Voices of
Lymphedema

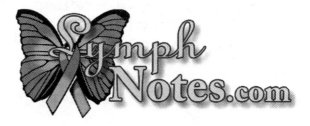

D0757111

Advanced praise for *Voices of Lymphedema*:

This book is a must read for all persons touched by lymphedema: persons with lymphedema, significant others, care givers, and members of the medical team. It provides a refreshing and informative perspective that is most often overlooked, that being the person living with or at risk for developing lymphedema.

This book communicates the emotional experience of lymphedema as no other. These amazing real life stories allowed you to look inside the life of persons living with this chronic disease. You will experience the gamut of emotions as you read this book.
Linda McGrath Boyle, PT, DPT, CLT-LANA

*In **Voices of Lymphedema**, the reader will find story after personal story of the difficulties and triumphs associated in living with primary and secondary lymphedema. This comprehensive book is very easy to read and provides practical advice that is readily applicable to everyday life. From the beginning, patients will be quickly assured of just how many voices exist in the lymphedema community and comforted in knowing that they are not alone. In addition, health care professionals will find this book to be a valuable and practical resource for patients who are dealing with a myriad of medical issues and who hope to one-day return to their prior level of activity.*
Mary Kathleen Kearse, PT, CLT-LANA

Wow. This easy to read book was a real "page turner." ... There were stories of inspiration and joy. There were stories that made me angry because folks had to suffer so much or so long before they got correct diagnosis and adequate therapy. The articles were heart-felt, uplifting and educational.

Overall, an excellent resource for lymphedema patients, therapists, and other health care practitioners. It's a book that should be required reading in all schools that turn out healthcare providers whether it's medical school, physical-occupational-massage therapy schools, nursing schools or courses that specialize in lymphedema management.
Kathryn McKillip Thrift, BS, CLT-LANA

Voices of Lymphedema

stories, advice, and inspiration from patients and therapists

edited by

Ann Ehrlich
Elizabeth McMahon, PhD
foreword by
Calina Burns

Lymph Notes
San Francisco

Voices of Lymphedema: stories, advice, and inspiration from patients
and therapists
© 2007 by Lymph Notes

Lymph Notes
2929 Webster Street
San Francisco, CA 94123 USA
www.LymphNotes.com   sales@lymphnotes.com

Notice of Rights
All rights reserved. No part of this book may be reproduced in any form or by any
means without prior permission of the publisher.

.

Notice of Liability
The information in this book is provided on an "as is" basis without warranty. It is sold
with the understanding that the publisher and authors are not engaged in providing
medical or other professional services. Neither the authors, nor Lymph Notes, shall
have any liability to any person or entity for any loss or damage caused or alleged to
be caused, indirectly or directly by the instructions contained in this book.

Trademarks
Lymph Notes is a registered trademark, LymphNotes.com, and the Lymph Notes logo
are trademarks of Lymph Notes. All product names and services identified throughout
this book are used in editorial fashion only; usage does not imply an endorsement or
affiliation.

ISBN 10: 0-9764806-5-4
ISBN 13: 978-0-9764806-5-5
Library of Congress Control Number: 2007936484
Publishing history—first edition, printing 1.00

Foreword

"We can create hope together and, together, we can make a difference!"

My name is Cheryl Calina Burns; I go by Calina. I am a secondary lymphedema patient and a member of the Board of Directors of the Lymphatic Research Foundation (LRF).

At 22 I had a radical hysterectomy and, several years later, developed lymphedema. I am now 46 and have lived with lymphedema for nearly 25 years.

Developing lymphedema was a devastating experience for me especially given the fact that I had started a modeling career. Terrified that my swelling would be noticed I promptly gave up my career and was quite depressed for sometime after.

Aside from the progression of my condition, there was very little medical or scientific information available. Treatment options were not made known to me for many years and the overall responses that I did get were negative with hopeless visions for the future.

Over the course of the following 15 years or so I lived with my condition as best I could. I worked very hard to keep the swelling concealed from employers, friends, dates, and so on.

This was quite difficult to do and I was often in pain and always uncomfortable. It was not until I found the Lymphatic Research Foundation (see page 221) at a conference that my life was transformed and hope for the future completely restored.

I have since come out of the closet with my condition and have decided that if I am going to have lymphedema then I must have it for a reason and must use it to effect change in any way I can through my service on the LRF board. I have stopped trying to hide my leg and I welcome the opportunity to talk about lymphedema and lymphatic diseases.

I take excellent care of myself and exercise regularly. I have found the more I exercise the better my leg does. I work out with weights and I rotate cardio machines to avoid too much repetitive motion. I do yoga, which I find is wonderful for lymphedema.

I do everything I want to do and refuse to allow my leg to limit me too much. I listen to my body and rest my leg when I need to. I go skiing, hiking, mountain biking, and play tennis; however, I do these things as a lymphedema patient and use good judgment at all times.

Although I wish there were a cure and would prefer not to have lymphedema, I have learned that one must forge ahead in spite of the obstacles we may face. Life must go on.

I have a tremendous sense of compassion for people with any malady or disability that I may not have developed had I not had lymphedema. I believe my experience has made me stronger as an individual.

It has become very important to me to do what I can to make a difference, not only in the area of lymphatic research, but in all areas of life. Wherever I can serve best is where I want and need to be.

I am so thrilled that someone has decided to write a positive book about the courage it takes to live with such a difficult condition. Lymphedema patients around the world need encouragement to learn how to control their malady rather than allow it to control them.

As patients, the sooner we all come to terms with our lymphedema, speak out and reach out, the sooner we can truly create change in terms of better care and possibly even a cure someday. We can create hope together and, together, we can all make a difference!

Calina Burns

Acknowledgements

This book exists because of the generosity and honesty of our contributors. The response to our request for stories was awe-inspiring and we thank each of you for caring enough to reach out and help others by sharing. Every contribution was valued and unique. We are more grateful than words can express to each of you.

Anonymous

Naomi Aaronson, MA OTR/L, CHT

David Adcock, PT, CLT

Ashley

Audrey

Mary Pat B.

Shelley Barlow

Suzi Beatie

Emily P. Bees

Betty

Brent

Tina Buddle

Calina Burns

CM

Kim Decker

Jackie Doss

Ann Ehrlich

Mary Essert, BA, ATRIC

Laurie Feest, OTR,CHT, LLCC

Lorelei Foss

Avid Gardner

Shirley Glick_

Judy Gloeckler

Joan Glunk, LMT, CLT

Shari Harper

Betty Harvey

Amy Hayes

Janet Hunt

Jane

Jeanette

Jennifer

Marcene Johansson

Carol L. Johnson, OTL, CLT-LANA

Anna Kellogg, OTR/L, CLT

Anna Kennedy

Keith

Nancy Kinzli, OT, CLT

Susan Klapper

Doris Laing, LMBT, CLT-LANA

Lymph Notes Members (10+)

Elizabeth McMahon, Ph.D.

Marty

Mary Anne McCarrick

Melanie

Bonnie Moats

Mom

Cheryl L. Morgan, CLT, MS, PhD

James Morrow, MT, CLT-LANA

Tracy Novak

Betty Oertel

Jayah Faye Paley

Ruthi Peleg, BPt, BS, CLT

Bonnie Pike

Barbara Pilvin

Liz Pomeroy, OTR, CLT-LANA

Melanie Posch, OTR-CLT

Karen Reckner

Remy

Emily Richter, RN, BSN, OCN

Renee Romero, RN, CLT-LANA

Rosa

Martha Ruppert

Judith Sedlak, PT, CLT

Elizabeth Shapiro, MS, OTR/L, CLT

Ya-Chen Tina Shih, PhD

Michelle Shippen

Georgia Spidle

Dixie Spiegel

Traci Spohn

Paula Stewart, MD, CLT-LANA

Fran Suran

Barbara Taylor

Josie Tenney

Lawrence L. Tretbar, MD, ScD, FACS

Alma Vinjé-Harrewijn, PT, CLT

Melba Walker

Mary D. Warren

Robert Weiss, MS

Joanne Young

In addition, we wish to specifically acknowledge Anna Kennedy and the Lymphovenous Association of Ontario for permitting us to summarize the "Lymph Listens" report.

We would also like to thank our reviewers for helping to ensure the high quality of this book:

George Bagby

Janet C. Baker

Linda McGrath Boyle, PT, DPT, CLT-LANA

Wendy Chaite, Esq.

Suzie Crocker

Laura Flint, PT, CLT

Tina Hammond, PTA, CLT-LANA

Cheri L. Hoskins, CCT

Mary Kathleen Kearse, PT, CLT-LANA

Anna Kellogg, OTR/L, CLT

Cheryl L. Morgan, CLT, MS, PhD

Ruthi Peleg, BPt, BS, CLT

JoAnn Rovig, LMT, CLT-LANA

Saskia R. J. Thiadens, RN

Kathryn McKillip Thrift, BS, CLT-LANA

Lawrence L. Tretbar, MD, ScD, FACS

Mary Vargo, MD

Robert Weiss, MS

We wish to publicly recognize and celebrate the courage it takes to live with lymphedema and the creative ways in which people meet this challenge. We want to thank those who care for lymphedema patients and who search for more effective treatment. Special acknowledgement is also due to the advocates working to make lymphedema care available to all who need it.

We would also like to acknowledge Barbara Delinsky's **Uplift**. We discovered this collection of tips and experiences shared by breast cancer survivors in early 2006 and were inspired to create a similar book for people with lymphedema.

On a personal note, we want to thank our husbands and families for their support, patience, and assistance throughout the process of bringing this book to fruition.

And finally, to our readers—we thank you for your time and attention. We hope each of you will share the inspiration, hope, and helpful information here and that you will spread the word so the message of this book will reach all who can benefit from reading it, whether patient, caregiver, or advocate.

Table of Contents

Contents in Brief

Contents in Detail

Introduction

Voices of Lymphedema provides a way for us to share and inspire. We want to celebrate the courageous, creative, resourceful people that make lemonade from that lemon—known as lymphedema—which life has handed them.

We chose stories to achieve these goals because stories are powerful. Facts are important, but dry facts do not convey the reality of human experience. Stories bring facts to life. The human voice speaking from the heart communicates the complex realities of living with lymphedema.

Our contributors speak eloquently and honestly about living with lymphedema. You will find everything from helpful hints to humor, from shared sympathy to calls for action.

So few people know about lymphedema that it has been called "a silent epidemic." The people speaking here are no longer willing to let that be the case. They want you to know what happens when lymphedema is undiagnosed or untreated for years. And they want you to know that effective treatment, by a trained therapist, can restore mobility and give people their lives back. Read about AZ, Betty, and Frances in Chapter 2—for a few examples.

We hope that our book will benefit several groups:

- *If you have lymphedema*, we want you to hear in a very personal way that you are not alone with your feelings and struggles. Our hope is that you feel encouraged, understood, supported, and less alone. Through practical tips and emotional encouragement, other people are reaching out to you in their own words.

- *If you do not have lymphedema*, these gripping, realistic, sometimes funny stories will give you a deeper respect and understanding of the reality of living with this condition. Our hope is that this understanding will help you to help others who have lymphedema—whether they are family members or friends, patients you treat, or those whom you are helping in a fight for insurance coverage, legislative change, or research and treatment.

- *If you are a medical professional*, we hope these stories from patients and other professionals will deepen your knowledge of the personal experience and impact of lymphedema as well as the benefits and necessity of effective treatment. Patients repeatedly voice the wish that their healthcare providers had told them about lymphedema and advised them about risk reduction. Perhaps you will be intrigued enough to learn more about the lymphatic system, lymphedema, and lymphedema treatment and to share this knowledge with fellow professionals.

Another goal for this book is to offer entertainment, encouragement, inspiration, and guidance. The people you will meet in this book talk about how creatively they fit treatment and self-care into their daily lives. You will find true-life stories of people's struggles and perseverance as they push to get a diagnosis, to find treatment, or to get reimbursement.

Learn how people just like you are raising public awareness of lymphedema and educating healthcare professionals, advocating for better treatment availability and reimbursement, and supporting legislative changes to protect the rights of people with lymphedema. Hopefully these stories will provide powerful ammunition and support all of these efforts.

We solicited stories from patients and professionals via the Lymph Notes website and our personal networks. Our contributors include men and women with primary and secondary lymphedema, primarily from the US and Canada. Some stories and names have been changed to respect the privacy of the authors or patients.

We've organized stories around these themes:

- **Unique and Universal Patient Stories** about the experience of living with lymphedema.

- **Stories from Professionals** about their experiences caring for patients, why they became therapists, and the rewards of their work.

- **Learning about Lymphedema,** with recommendations for obtaining information, getting a diagnosis, and finding treatment, plus answers to frequently asked questions.

- **Activities** enjoyed by people with lymphedema and suggestions on adapting your activities if you have lymphedema.

- **Travel** stories and tips from active travelers with lymphedema.

- **Solutions** to common problems related to living with lymphedema.

- **Self-Care Tips** from therapists and patients.

- **Humor**, frankly there is not a lot of lymphedema humor, but we hope these pieces trigger a chuckle or a rueful grin of recognition.

- **Support Groups,** ways for people to come together in person and online to help each other including examples of some successful groups and tips for starting your own group.

- **Outreach to Medical Professionals** to help them understand lymphedema and its treatment.

- **Reimbursement Policy Issues,** information and tools for advocacy.

- **Postscript** summarizing some of the lessons offered here.

- **Appendix** includes an explanation of lymphedema, a lymphedema glossary, warning signs for lymphedema and infections, lymphedema resources, and more. *If you are not familiar with lymphedema or lymphedema treatment, you might want to read the Appendix first.*

As you will see in this book we, as a community, face three related challenges:

- **Education**: medical professionals and patients with, or at risk for, lymphedema need better awareness of what lymphedema is, its frequency, its diagnosis, the availability of effective treatments, and standards of care for treatment. We also need better evidence of treatment effectiveness (that goes beyond the anecdotes we present here), comprehensive disease management programs for lymphedema—similar to diabetes management programs—with an emphasis on treatment that prevents infections and disability and maximizes quality of life, and more effective treatment options.

- **Reimbursement**: is a tangled cluster of challenges—

  o Lack of healthcare coverage and limited coverage is a larger policy issue and not specific to lymphedema. Lymphedema makes this problem more critical because most lymphedema patients, especially those with secondary lymphedema, have multiple medical conditions.

  o Coverage that does not reimburse lymphedema therapy at all, or sets unrealistically low limits on the number of treatments. Better coverage involves the issues discussed under education above, plus more appropriate diagnostic, treatment, and billing codes.

○   Lack of adequate coverage, even in the more generous plans, for all the bandaging supplies, compression garments, and compression devices required for effective care. The cost of these supplies and devices places a severe financial burden on many patients.

•   **Therapist Availability**: the shortage of qualified therapists relates, in part, to the education and reimbursement issues outlined above but a recent development has made a bad situation even worse. Medicare (and many other payers that follow Medicare policies) recently decided that they will only reimburse physical and occupational therapists for providing lymphedema treatment. Massage therapists and nurses will not be reimbursed, even if they have specialized training and experience in treating lymphedema. The irony of this move is that most of the pioneers and thought leaders in lymphedema treatment in the US are nurses and massage therapists!

Lymphedema is too important not to be talked about. We encourage you to join us in declaring, "We will not allow lymphedema to be a silent epidemic any longer!" and, if you are so inclined, working to change policies and laws.

Share your story with us. We invite you personally to e-mail us at Ann@LymphNotes.com and send us your own stories or tips for possible inclusion in future editions. We would also love to hear your feedback and reactions. We look forward to hearing from you.

Now sit back, keep reading, and enjoy!

Best wishes, Ann and Elizabeth

Chapter 1

Unique and Universal Patient Stories

Editors' Note: We begin with stories that reflect many of the common experiences with lymphedema. Each story has aspects that are individual and unique, and each reflects aspects of the lymphedema experience that are universal.

You will notice certain themes that occur in these stories and resurface throughout the book. For example, one theme is that of noticing what works and building on that awareness. Noticing what works can involve noticing early signs of positive change, monitoring lymphedema and looking for patterns, or discovering what actions make a difference and then repeating them.

In so many of the stories, the focus is on problem-solving, progress, and successes. You will find great ideas as others with lymphedema share what works for them. For more ideas, see chapters 4-7 on Activities, Travel, Solutions to Common Problems, and Self-Care Tips. The Postscript pulls together the lessons from these stories and talks about effective coping.

Lymphedema is a challenge, but we generally grow more through challenging or difficult times than we do through easy, comfortable times. As the saying goes, "Every problem comes bearing a gift in its hands."

Throughout this book, you will find examples of creating positives out of the negative of lymphedema. As you reflect on the ways the people in this book have grown in knowledge, acceptance, spirituality, you may recognize ways that you have grown because of, or in spite of, your lymphedema.

Reading Betty's story (page 36) helps put living with lymphedema in perspective. Life isn't perfect, but we've come a long way—and together we can make things even better.

We hope that reading these stories encourages and inspires you. We hope you resonate to the stories here and in the chapters to come. We thank every contributor for sharing their insights, their knowledge and their experiences. This book is composed of a "chorus" of individual voices.

Lymphedema, a Gift of My Breast Cancer

"Spread the word about lymphedema to others— particularly those working with, or facing, cancer."

Editors' Note: Like so many of the wonderful people you will meet between the covers of this book, Fran shares her experience in the hope that "change will happen and it will be an easier path" for those with lymphedema.

My name is Fran. I had breast cancer and I have lymphedema—one of the gifts of my breast cancer. Thanks for inviting me to share my story. Lymphedema is unique for each person. I can only talk from my perspective.

The first time I heard about lymphedema was through the informal women's network. Several women who had already done the breast cancer tour of duty alerted me to lymphedema and also mentioned that finding information and treatment would be difficult, particularly within the medical community. They were right.

The top cancer hospitals in this city (Toronto, Canada) offered no information, help, or treatment. Most doctors were not aware of it. There is very little research for this chronic, progressive condition. It doesn't appeal to the drug companies for funding and so far, no magic pills to cure it. Many cancer websites and organizations including the Canadian Breast Cancer Foundation hadn't heard of it. The States are easily 10 years ahead of us on lymphedema, and places like Europe and Australia are even farther ahead.

As with the rest of my breast cancer course, I empowered myself, I researched, I asked questions, I became educated and I advocated for myself. When I asked about lymphedema, my first surgeon dismissed my questions and told me not to worry about lymphedema, because it *"hardly ever happens,"* and if it did there was nothing you could do about it anyway.

My current surgeon told me that I was his first patient with lymphedema. From what I have experienced and heard, these are typical responses from the medical community. Though statistics are hard to find, that *"hardly ever happens"* is in the 20 to 30% range and radiation of the lymph node area can increase the risk of lymphedema by 50%.

Through the informal women's network I was directed to physiotherapists (physical therapists) specially trained in lymphedema.

I went for a consult before my surgery, and after my surgery had preventative therapy throughout my chemo and radiation. Once lymph nodes have been removed the onset of lymphedema can occur at any time, even years after your surgery and cancer treatments. That's why it's especially important for health care practitioners, and particularly family physicians, to be made aware of lymphedema.

My lymphedema—which is in my arm, my breast, and my trunk—started during my radiation. As I was aware of lymphedema, I could do something about it and deal with it. Early detection, education, and treatment are important for lymphedema management. Patients and health care practitioners should not dismiss, but pay attention to early signs of lymphedema such as aching, tingling and heaviness which are often present before the swelling.

Lymphedema has changed my life dramatically. Even though it has taken awhile, I feel that I have embraced and accepted both the emotional aspects and physical limitations of my lymphedema. It is a constant balancing act with a lot of trial and error. I listen to my body. If I go overboard, I pay. I rest often. I have given up many things I really enjoy, that aggravate my lymphedema. I have made many changes and accommodations in my daily life in order to manage my lymphedema and to try to improve my quality of life.

For example, if possible, driving and taking the subway in off-peak hours and driving with a pillow under my affected arm. Rearranging cupboards so there is less reaching, breaking tasks into smaller chunks so as to not over do. Also I avoid carrying heavy items such as a purse, laptop computer, briefcase, knapsack, or groceries on my affected side. For my purse I use a fanny pack that also doubles as an arm rest. I use a headset for the telephone. For first line defense in case of cuts, I always carry a lymphedema emergency purse kit with alcohol wipes, topical antibiotic, and band-aids.

I don't cook as much and serve more *"homemade in someone else's kitchen."* I try to avoid repetitive motions with my arm such as being on the computer too long, shoveling snow, vacuuming, scrubbing pots, playing tennis, and lifting weights. I try to exercise regularly, in moderation, and do yoga.

I try to be more flexible and less stressed and not worry about things that are not under my control—like moody teenagers and the weather. Humidity, heat and low pressure particularly affect me. As I was reviewing these notes I knew that the weather was changing. I felt heaviness, discomfort, pain and swelling in my arm, my trunk and my breast. My body is a very accurate forecaster, better than the professional weather forecasters!

This has all been very new ground for a previous Type A person. I follow the regular treatment program called Combined Decongestive Therapy. This includes weekly lymph drainage massage from a specially trained therapist, wearing compression garments (Bellisse bra, custom sleeve and glove), doing self-massage at home, and becoming educated and practicing safe lymphedema management.

I take preventative steps such as: not having blood pressure or any injections in my affected arm; and avoiding hot showers, saunas, hot tubs and sunburns. I wear gloves to wash dishes, do housework, and garden. I wear compression garments, and a Medic Alert bracelet for lymphedema. I try to avoid any break in the skin on my affected side. This includes scraps, injections, insect bites, pet scratches, or paper cuts that could cause a life-threatening infection and result in a visit to the ER for IV antibiotics and a hospital stay. Should this happen, I have to hope the ER staff has heard of lymphedema.

It has been said that *"Education dispels fear."* Personally I feel so empowered knowing what I do and being able to make my choices and improve my quality of life. This is why I feel it is so important to educate others and raise awareness about lymphedema. Through my involvement as a board member of the Lymphovenous Association of Ontario, I hear too many preventable lymphedema horror stories. It is difficult to get a lymphedema diagnosis or to find information, treatment, and garments. The treatments and garments are expensive and are minimally covered by the government and most private insurance plans. The garments are unattractive, hot and uncomfortable – often I can't wait to rip them off. Finding clothing that fits is a challenge. Living with lymphedema is on going, time-consuming, frustrating, and expensive and a constant reminder of your cancer.

AND IT IS FOR THE REST OF YOUR LIFE.

Lymphedema is just one of many cancer leftovers or gifts that fall into the void of post cancer care. In fact, the recent Canadian Breast Cancer Foundation Study *"Toward Kinder Care"* (www.upfrontproject.ca) highlights this. I continue to take the opportunity to talk to as many people as possible in the hope that change will happen and it will be an easier path for the increasing number of survivors who follow. You too can spread the word about lymphedema — particularly those working with or facing any cancer in which lymph node removal surgery is involved.

Fran Suran

Fran is a Director of the Lymphovenous Association of Ontario (see page 223) and a Peer Mentor for the Breast Cancer Survivorship Program at the Princess Margaret Hospital, Toronto, Canada.

My Adventures with Lymphedema

"I am not about to let lymphedema run my life!"

Editors' Note: This free-form poem by Jayah captures the ups and downs, the hopes and fears of cancer and lymphedema (LE). It is a triumphant journey.

Breast Cancer, drats
Chemo, double drats
Radiation, sigh
Lymphedema? PANIC! TILT!!

Was it just the last straw syndrome or the reality that this is a condition I'd dreaded and would have to manage for the rest of my life?

After 3 surgeries to get clear margins and all the treatment(s), LE just seemed like a bit TOO MUCH.

Get a GRIP. I knew what to do.
I had been learning my self drainage, had sought treatment before ever noticing that first swelling.
I had taken the Upledger Lymphatic Drainage Course years ago as part of my continuing education as a massage therapist.
I knew about the lymphatic system, about drainage – I was ahead of the game.
I would not get LE,
RIGHT.

One day in June, at the end of a short recovery hike, I noticed swelling in my right arm.
Denial.
Anger.
Rush to the LE therapist. Please tell me this is not LE.

Fast forward.
Actually, rewind.
I noticed a lump in October.
My GYN said, *"It's nothing, I can't feel anything."*
Three months later, I went back.
He said the same.
I sat up and said, but I can see it.
His response was—are you ready for this? *"Oh my God."*

Nice thing to hear from a doc, huh?

He got me into see a breast cancer surgeon in three days.
Two days later, at 5 pm on Friday afternoon, I got the call—it's breast cancer.
The following Tuesday, I had a lumpectomy.
Two days later, January 30, 2003, my long time live-in companion married me so I'd have better insurance.
Instead of running away screaming (like the ex-speaker of the House), he ran towards me.
A scientist, a researcher, an advocate—my Bob.
Thus began a year of fighting.

Now fast forward to LE troubles, and troubles they were.
I sought care, I sought information, I sought treatment.
I wanted to continue my activities and my work.
My two favorite activities both involved my arms – sea kayaking and hiking WITH POLES.
Whether it was denial, stubbornness or just plain ignorance, I was not about to let LE run my life.

I became the fibrosis queen.
I would get treatment and two days later my arm would be firm again… not just swollen, but firm.
A top quality LE therapist could not figure it out. She had been treating LE for 25 years (rather unusual in this game) and had never seen anyone like me.

Another rewind—this experience became normal for me.
Whenever my surgeon told me there was a 3% chance or a 5% chance of something – that was me. I learned to ignore those small percentages to prevent total devastation.

So here I was, the fibrosis queen, trying to figure out ways to continue exercising, enjoying life and connecting with my buddies.

My top quality therapist was not on my insurance so I searched around and started seeing other people.
I quickly realized there is a huge variance in the quality of care.

My first experience was with a therapist in a major hospital. She had a cold and refused to wear a mask. She told me she did not do hands on work. A LE therapist who does not do hands on work sounds to me like an oxymoron. Crossed her off my list.

Another major hospital had a whole LE department—that was where I was bandaged so badly that I developed new and significant swelling in my fingers. When I complained (what did I know at that time about wrapping? Very little in fact and depended on her to know her job), she unwrapped and re-bandaged me. The next day I had a whole new set of problems (that took months to resolve).

After about 18 different therapists, I knew what to look for. I understood there were different techniques and that each technique—or school—had its advantages and uses. I found a massage therapist who was doing a study. A Vodder school practitioner, she was offering a special arrangement for the study so I had treatment twice a week during radiation. Since radiation can often worsen LE, this proved to be inspired.

Still, though, I was the fibrosis queen.

Major rewind.

I created the only comprehensive education on how to use poles for hiking. Trekking poles help people achieve better balance, endurance, posture and strength—while enjoying the outdoors. As a result of this and the seminars and training I was doing, I received a referral to a man who changed my life.

An ex-trauma surgeon, turned osteopath, Joel had become disenchanted (or tired) with cutting and wanted to heal more naturally. He lived on a farm way up in the hills of north Sonoma County (quite a drive for me from Pacifica, California). A tractor had run over his back and he was told he'd never walk again. Determined (can you say Type A?), he contacted me and I helped him walk with poles.

Joel saw what I was going thru and he thought he could, in turn, help me. He treated me and, VOILA, the fibrosis got better.
Here's the problem: MLD is gentle, fibrosis work is deep and undoes some of the good work that is needed for creating the collateral vessels.
Joel showed me how an osteopathic machine, called a percussor, could do deep work gently.
It was a miracle.

I plunked down $500 for the machine and another $500 to learn how to use it and it was the best $1000 I ever spent.
I could now treat myself for the firming without damaging the gentle vessels.

Overall, I spent about 4-5 hours per day for over 6 months.
Fighting, managing LE became my full time job.

I would tape a silly show, watch it (fast forwarding thru the commercials) and that's exactly the amount of time it took me to do my MLD.

When I told my radiation oncologist about my horror stories and how I'd finally (after dreadful experiences and much sorrow) found solutions, he recommended I speak with a woman who coordinated the breast cancer patients' care for the hospital. After several attempts, she one day answered the phone.

After about a 20 minute recital of the saga I experienced, she suggested we discuss starting a LE Group.

I was adamant, I did not want to start a support group. I was solely interested in education, resources and exercise.
Thus began our LEEG - Lymphedema Education & Exercise Group.
We now have three top therapists (and I know they're top because I have been treated by each of them and I know what to look for) and me. We run the group every month. It's free to anyone with or at risk for LE. We help primary, secondary, anyone. We help people understand, manage and prevent LE.

For information on resources, please visit my (always a work in progress) website: www.AdventureBuddies.NET
Do not settle.
Work at managing LE

My sister told me something one day as I was telling her about MY lymphedema. She said—don't own it. I learned to call it the LE, not MY LE. Somehow that helped. It distanced me and made it less a part of me.

Currently I do not wear a sleeve. Yes, I travel with one, but do not wear it. My night and day wear are packed away in case I need them, and at the first sign of swelling, I'm on it, doing my MLD. I get treatment about eight times a year for prevention and to facilitate flow, plus it feels good.

Life is full, LE is in the background – not forgotten, but understood and managed.

Jayah Faye Paley

Editors' Reminder: Please remember that appropriate treatment will vary from person to person. Check any specific treatment advice with your health care team before following it.

Back to School

"What happened? Did your lunch slide down to your feet?"

Editors' Note: Ashley shares her experience as a teenager facing high school with primary lymphedema.

I was born with primary lymphedema . Most of the time while I was growing up it seemed pretty normal for me to have to go for treatments, wear compression garments, and all of that "stuff." But now all of that has changed!

This year I started high school. I hate the idea of being different. Compression hose do not make a fashion statement!

Some of the other kids think I'm weird because I've got this "fat leg" and I get comments like, *"What happened? Did your lunch slide down to your feet?"* The others think this is funny, and I try to laugh too—but it hurts.

And then there's my mom. She still insists that I keep up the lymphedema routine. I'm so tired of it. I want to quit. I just want to be "normal." On top of that she keeps after me to keep my weight down to get out and ride my bike for exercise. (Bike riding bike is fun but I'm not about to tell her that.)

Like all of the other new students, I had a "getting to know you" interview with a school counselor. She has a reputation for being a really cool lady who listens. So I told her about the lymphedema and how I was feeling.

To my amazement she came around the desk, slid up the pants leg of her slacks and said, *"You mean compression garments like this?"* Wow, she has lymphedema too! Seems she developed it after cancer surgery. The cause is different, but we still share the same problems.

She gave me some good tips on how to cope with "being different," reassured me that as others got to know me they would come to know me as a person, and invited me to come back to talk anytime I wanted. This has been a big help.

Ashley

With a Happy Heart and an Altered Body

" I am better, stronger and more resilient than I ever was before."

Editors' Note: Shelley sent us her story with this introduction, "I came across your paperwork and would like to share my story about my health situation and challenges in the hope that my story might help others."

Back in August of 2005, I was diagnosed with Inflammatory Breast Cancer. Within the week, I gave my work notice of my situation, saw the oncologist, and began chemo. I was officially off work for one year. I teach in a childcare center with 16 preschoolers and have been in the field for 25 years. Being in childcare, I chose not to have children, so being off for a year was like my maternity leave without the child in tow. It was real difficult for me to just stop, focus on my health—and for once in my life—tend to me and not others.

I had eight chemo treatments and finished on January 25, 2006. Then, in March, I had both breasts removed because I did not want to have a recurring problem in future years.

I had my surgery on a Friday and, by the next Monday I began to have swelling in my left arm. I had read about lymphedema and the possibility of me having it. Initially I thought it was okay. It was neat how the body is connected, how the dents in my arm took so long to push out, how my fingerprints lasted on my arm a bit. I celebrated my new life with a luncheon for 69 of my closest friends including those who had come to my rescue when I was down and out.

Then I underwent 25 radiation treatments finishing in July of 2006. After my radiation, I tended to my arm and now know the lasting features that I am living with presently will be a lifetime problem and challenge.

It was my goal to return to work in September when the new school year began, along with all of my new students. With that in mind, I worked out at Curves to build up my strength and endurance to help me get through my day, as well as the hour that I drive to and from work each day.

I attended the Cookstown Wellness Centre in Ontario for massages and care. I also have compression garments and a hand glove. I have been wearing the arm sleeve regularly but have the glove just in case I overdo yard work or exert too much energy, causing swelling.

My hand seems to be under control as I do self-massages each evening to keep everything in check. Now it is May, and I feel wonderful. My strength is back and I listen to what my body tells me.

My mind, soul and body have been through a lot. I came out of surgery with two lovely scars as mementos of what I have been through. I can hide them under my clothing. My left arm is a different story.

When I was still at home, my arm was still in hiding. When I returned to work, I was asked a lot of questions. The parents and the children were curious, the bank teller, the drive-through person who I see each morning for coffee all wanted to know how I had hurt myself. If they only knew what had happened and what a loaded question they were asking of me!

I quickly had to come up with a line to explain why I was wearing the sleeve and not make them feel embarrassed for the asking. I told them my arm was swelling from a recent surgery that I had had. They still wanted to know more. When I told them more, their mouth dropped open and they didn't know what to say.

For the longest time, I felt ashamed of the way I looked. No breasts. Sleeve on my arm. Grey hair that used to be blonde and puffy. Fatter, as I had put on 40 pounds due to chemo, steroids, good eating, and being on Herceptin for a year. My new breasts were heavy and uncomfortable. Putting them on felt like I was strapping on a heavy fanny pack filled with coins. Dish gloves were required as a donning aid to pull the compression sleeve over my swollen and heavy arm.

This was my new look that I had to get used to seeing in the mirror each and every day. I used to wear contacts, now I wear bifocals. My feet grew another shoe size while I was ill. There were so many changes to deal with both physically and emotionally. The fall was a challenge for me and then we gradually progressed into winter.

During the winter months, I was able to cover up my arm. I noticed that all my clothing was tight and always pulled in the shoulder area. My older clothing had to be replaced with newer, bigger, and wider sizes that would accommodate my new body.

Long gone is the pretty, preppy clothing I once wore. Now, I wear a man's t-shirt to have enough room in the arm without any pulling. Not being able to wear women's clothing makes you feel even worse as you feel you are loosing more of your identity. Not only are the breasts gone, the arm is big, your clothes are big and your old self is gone, never to return in this lifetime. It was difficult to resort to men's clothing. They just don't make them real pretty like women's!!! So the feminine side of me is gone and I have lost more than breasts and a skinny arm.

Now it is May and here it is Mother's Day. By now I am feeling better about myself, and my situation. I guess I just needed some time to find the new me, the different-looking me, the better me. I may look different on the outside and people view me in a different light. I know the real me is inside and know the trials and challenges I have endured.

I am better, stronger and more resilient than I ever was before. I am happy to be alive, to have lymphedema therapists to help keep my body and soul in check, to have a medical team that cares for me on an ongoing basis, and to be here another year to share my story with others. My body is an educational tool. I will continue to share my challenges and successes with others in hopes they can rise to the occasion and share their story with others too.

With a happy heart and an altered body,

Shelley Barlow

My Journey from Parasites to Fashion

"When faced with lymphedema, I did what I have always done before. That is to make the best of the situation and add a little fun."

Editors' Note: Kim's story talks about the ways she went about finding solutions to the challenges of lymphedema.

My name is Kim Decker and my educational background is in the biology of parasites. But it is funny where life takes you and this is the story of my journey from parasites to fashion.

I was diagnosed with breast cancer and developed lymphedema in my arm after completing chemotherapy but before going through radiation. I was frustrated to learn that this is a chronic condition—one I will have to pay attention to the rest of my life; however, I am grateful to have found a physical therapist that specializes in lymphedema treatment.

When faced with lymphedema, I did what I have always done before. That is to make the best of the situation and add a little fun. For the first year and a half of treatment, I wore a compression sleeve all the time. It was during this time that I began creating arm covers to enhance the appearance of compression sleeves. This "hobby" eventually turned into the business known as a Slice of Fashion LLC which specializes in the design and fabrication of arm covers to jazz up compression garments.

As I learned more, it became increasingly obvious that lymphedema is not well understood and that research on it is sorely needed and severely under funded. Therefore, as my business grows, I hope to donate some of the profits to lymphedema research.

Kim Decker,
Founder of Slice of Fashion LLC
www.sliceoffashion.com

Editors' Note: Continuing the theme of poetry to express the experience of living with lymphedema, Kim shares two haiku. Our wish for you is that the good days outnumber the bad ones. We hope these stories give you the support and suggestions you need to do so.

Day by Day with Lymphedema

On a Bad Day
Swollen like sausage
Blotchy pain constant vigil
For the rest of life

On a Good Day
My arm, part of me
I create and live with joy
I am here with smile

Kim Decker

What I Have Learned from Lymphedema So Far

"I try to maintain a 'culture of wellness' in our home"

Editors' Note: Joanne gives her overview of living with lymphedema. Which of her experiences, insights, and ways of coping reflect your own experience?

Lymphedema is both feared and dreaded by cancer survivors as a potential secondary outcome of their treatment. It appears to me that the most positive aspect to this situation is that an increasing number of patients have some awareness that lymphedema exists, although they may not actually know much about it.

In that way, I was fortunate during my first encounter with cancer, as I had not even *heard* of lymphedema—and therefore only had to concentrate on recovery, without the added worry of developing some other condition. In 1992, I was diagnosed with cervical adenocarcinoma and within days of receiving the news met with a team of doctors for staging and a treatment proposal. At the staging appointment, I was extremely relieved to be told that the best plan for my care would be to have a radical hysterectomy.

What I wanted, more than anything, was for them to remove the cancer at the earliest time possible. At the time of my diagnosis, my daughter had just turned eight years old, and my only sibling—a sister eighteen months older than myself with whom I had been very close—had passed away suddenly six months earlier. Our family had been living in a state of shock since her death at only thirty-seven years old, and my sudden health crisis was another cause for upheaval. Needless to say, I was terrified to have a diagnosis of cancer suddenly enter my life.

When the surgeon explained that part of the radical surgery involved removing lymph nodes from the inguinal area in order to ensure no spread of the cancer, I was totally ignorant of any potential complications. It would not have occurred to me to even ask, as all I knew was that this wonderful person and everyone there knew exactly what to do to help me. My focus was on getting through the process and resuming our normal family life as quickly as possible. On our fourteenth wedding anniversary, I had my surgery.

Never having had major surgery before, I had no idea about what to expect while recovering. Post-surgery and in the weeks following, I had aches and pains in my legs. I was noticeably puffy all over. Every physical anomaly that I experienced, I attributed to the challenges of a post-surgical body repairing itself.

Several weeks afterwards I could not believe how dramatically my body had changed. I had much bigger legs. I had always been rather slim and now I looked very different. My surgeon told me perhaps I wasn't being active enough. I had never had large legs and really didn't agree that I was being inactive. However, I felt rather challenged by his remark and immediately began biking 10 miles a day through the hills of the Niagara escarpment. I became obsessed with biking. I joined a gym and added weight training and aerobics to my daily fitness routine. Then I decided that the fittest people I knew were runners. I began to train, working up to a five-mile daily run, with a long run of 7-10 miles on weekends.

Neither my surgeon, nor my family doctor, ever suggested the possibility of lymphedema. My ankles would be conspicuously swollen at night, but most of the swelling would be down by the morning. My doctor sent me for tests, as there were times when I had quite a lot of pain. The tests indicated nothing wrong, and I began to really think I was 'losing it.' The initial symptoms of lymphedema can be very transitory.

Then it all came to a head. I am self-employed and had a high-pressure deadline for work, and the weather was extremely hot and humid. In the late afternoon of this scorching, stressful day—knowing I would be working late into the night—I decided to go for a long run to decompress and collect my thoughts for the coming few hours. So I did about an eight-mile run. After my run and a hot shower, I felt pretty good—but over the next several hours the skin on my right foot and ankle got tighter and tighter. I couldn't believe my eyes. My toes were like little sausages. My foot was a puffy fat pillow. My ankle was gone. I thought I must have somehow injured myself on my run. Rather than going away over night, the swelling got worse. The next day, my regular doctor being away, I went to see a different doctor. She looked at my leg and my foot and, after asking me about my medical history she stated in a no-nonsense way *"That's lymphedema."*

Not knowing a single thing about it, I waited for her to write the prescription or suggest physio or whatever would fix it. Then she stated matter-of-factly that I was *'going to have to live with it.'* She recommended going to the drugstore and getting an off-the-shelf knee-high compression stocking, to be worn daily, and elevating the leg a couple of times per day. I was in disbelief about the entire revelation. However, I did what she said. I immediately got the stocking; although I must admit finding the time to elevate the leg was a bit challenging. Not knowing any better, I continued to run almost daily. Even though it hurt, I did what came naturally at that point—run 'through' the pain. Needless to say, my ankle and foot continued to grow over the next several months. As well, I was in considerable pain, especially at the beginning of a run, until the ankle 'loosened up,' and then again later in the day when my leg, ankle, and foot were at their most swollen.

No one warned me that the swelling would eventually begin to harden. Gradually I realized that my leg and foot were becoming quite deformed. It became increasingly evident to me when I could barely tie my running shoe on my right foot. My edema was permanently firm and non-pitting. My regular doctor prescribed a diuretic for me—to help try to reduce the edema. Although well intentioned, the doctor apparently didn't realize that a diuretic is contra-indicated for lymphedema because even if the fluid is removed from the interstitial tissue all the protein-rich material that hardens over time is left behind.

Around that time, the Internet was just becoming more accessible – otherwise I would have had earlier access to up-to-date information. Many times, in attempts to solve the mystery of what was happening to me, I had gone to the library in our small town and consulted the Merck manual but its information on lymphedema was minimal and consisted of about 6 lines.

Fortunately, my husband went online to see what he could find out about lymphedema. He found a report of a study at Harvard in which lymphedema patients had been treated with a form of massage and compression therapy. There were before and after pictures of patients illustrating changes in their limbs following treatment. I took a print-out of the article to the surgeon and said, *"I want to go there."*

It was actually his nurse who told me that there was somebody at Scarborough General Hospital who might be able to help me. She gave me the phone number of Catherine Cotton, a physiotherapist (Editor's Note: the American term is physical therapist) who had done Complete Decongestive Therapy (CDT) training in the Vodder method. CDT is an intensive program of manual lymph drainage and compression therapy. Cathy Cotton assessed me and told me she thought she could help me, and for several weeks, I went everyday to the hospital for a one-hour treatment of manual lymph drainage and compression bandaging.

During that time, Cathy gave me lots of information about lymphedema. She also made me smile when she told me she 'had only hands, not wands.' To me the effects of manual lymph drainage and compression therapy were magical; not only was my leg much smaller, but my ankle had reappeared with vastly increased flexibility. My leg also felt much better from my toes up—less burning, less aching.

Following my course of treatment with Cathy, I had a good summer—even though my new compression garment took some getting used to. At the gym I took up rowing, a good upper body aerobic exercise, which took some of the strain off my leg, although I continued to walk (not run) and I maintained my regimen of weight training. My right leg maintained its new shape well over that summer. It wasn't the same leg it once had been, before lymphedema, but it looked and certainly felt a lot better. I went for a manual lymph drainage treatment on that leg once a month and wore my new custom-fitted toe-to-hip legging on my right leg every day over my wrapped sausage toes.

In November of 1999, at the age of 44, I had my first mammogram. I was surprised to be called back, needless to say, and then had an ultrasound, followed by a breast biopsy. I found out I had breast cancer, and early in January 2000, I had a modified radical mastectomy on my left side. I asked my surgeon beforehand if I could have a sentinel node biopsy rather than the usual chain of axillary nodes removed and she asked why 'we' would do that.

I explained that I had lower limb lymphedema from previous surgery for cancer. She told me, *"Oh no, we never see lymphedema anymore,"* and she seemed to think it was odd that I felt there could be any connection between lymphedema in my leg and the potential for developing it in my arm following more surgery.

Although I had no way of knowing it at the time, I now know that she responded that way because in many instances patients are out of the surgeon's care by the time they develop lymphedema. Being anxious to deal with the situation and knowing of her skill as a surgeon, I went ahead with the surgery she proposed, and started chemo. I must interject that in the midst of chemo we moved from our home of sixteen years to a farm—just to add a bit more upheaval to our lives! We had already become immersed in the process before my diagnosis.

Later that year when some friends were taking me out for lunch, I stepped from the car into an unpaved, uneven parking lot, turning my left ankle. By that evening, my lower left leg was aching and growing and the edema was moving upward.

I now have lymphedema from the waist down. I also have it in my left arm—relatively mildly. Needless to say, I treat that arm like gold. Whenever I have a twinge or tightness, I do a bit of self-massage. I elevate my arm like a semaphore signal the moment it aches or feels heavy. I continue to lift weights, although very lightly and with many reps, as it makes sense to me, knowing that muscle contractions help to move lymph. Having good musculature in the arm 'at risk,' to me, means greater strength and less likelihood of straining the arm, which could cause more lymphedema. I am very certain that not lifting weights makes my arm feel worse. If I had some other readily accessible form of upper body exercise, such as swimming, I might be tempted to forgo the weight lifting, but I feel it is better than nothing. Furthermore, I have recently seen a couple of articles suggesting that bench pressing might actually be good for lymphedema sufferers. All I know is, it is good for me! Because I have a good chance of developing more severe lymphedema on that side, I have not considered breast reconstruction surgery to be an option. Nor do I wear a prosthesis or anything that might irritate the sensitive skin on that side.

In October of 2000, I went to my first Lymphovenous Association of Ontario (LAO) Conference. It had taken me from the fall of 1992, until the late summer of 1998, to get a diagnosis of lymphedema and following that until the spring of 1999 to get treatment. Although I believe they were doing their best, I had felt extremely let down by my doctors. As well, while I had been fortunate to have my first round of intensive therapy done at a hospital and therefore covered by the provincial health plan, I now was on my own in terms of the expense of treating and maintaining control of my lymphedema.

I hoped that joining an organization like the LAO might help me to obtain further answers and I also felt it was important to participate in an organization that was trying to make inroads for lymphedema patients. At the Annual General Meeting, then-President Rob Girvan informed the delegates that the Board of Directors needed a Secretary. I was definitely interested in helping out and suddenly that seemed like a good place to start. So it was in the role of Secretary that I began going to Board meetings.

Then, as there are now, there were many issues to address, and much work to do to raise awareness of lymphedema amongst patients, healthcare workers and the general public. As well, there is the on-going challenge of funding for the Lymphovenous Association itself—obviously critical to keeping the organization alive. As it turned out, I was on the Board for five years in a variety of roles including two years as President. I left the Association as of November 2005, primarily for health reasons.

I am a professional artist, and continue to work as a freelance writer and illustrator from my home. Being self-employed, for the most part I am able to set my own hours. I feel an increasing drive to express that there is far more to me than my struggle with lymphedema, which has such an impact on my life. Other than the requirement to include some physical activity in my schedule every few hours, my enjoyment of my work allows me to be in a place where my lymphedema is of little or no consequence. That said, I cannot spend the time working that I once could; sitting for many hours, or even standing in front of an easel, definitely leads to an increase in my discomfort and edema.

Some people seem surprised to learn that through all of my challenges with regard to my health, I have never, never, thought *"Why me?"* To me, the question is, *"Why NOT me?"* In other words, why would I consider myself so exceptional as to be immune from any of these ultimately human things? It is easy enough to consider that there are worse conditions and far more suffering in the world. However, I do not want you to think that I am a 'Pollyanna' about all this.

There are times I am angry, sometimes at a rolling boil, actually. I get angry when I hear yet another story about the lack of information and support some patients get from their doctors, as well as when I hear of people who cannot afford treatment. I get exasperated when I see that lymphedema is never mentioned in any of the glamorous, high-profile fundraising events around breast cancer, when we know the risk factor for breast cancer patients for developing lymphedema over their lifetime is between 10 and 40 percent, with some estimates ranging as high as 60%.

Like everyone else, I am happy to celebrate the survivorship of cancer patients. However for cancer patients who subsequently develop lymphedema, moving on is much more challenging. They have been treated for a life-threatening illness, and their treatment has left them with an uncomfortable, restrictive, chronic condition they will have to manage for the rest of their lives, *with little or no support from the very people who were instrumental in provoking its onset.*

As many of us know only too well, in many cases they are left pretty well on their own—trying to find more answers, often struggling to afford treatment, dealing on a daily basis with fallout from the very procedures that helped save their lives. It is as though they have become orphans of the healthcare system.

Given that we know that any cancer survivor who has had lymph nodes removed surgically or radiation therapy is at risk for developing lymphedema over their lifetime, surely a small percentage of funds from what appears to be a plethora of gala fundraisers for all types of cancer could be directed to a Canadian facility dedicated to treating lymphedema. While some cancer centers now have lymphedema clinics, and that is an improvement over having nothing at all, they do not address the need for treatment. One clinic is offering four treatments but considering that each patient should ideally have CDT followed by a weekly hour-long MLD treatment, it is not enough.

In Germany and Austria, each lymphedema patient is entitled to two sessions, each of two weeks duration, of fully funded live-in treatment at clinics dedicated to treating lymphedema *annually*. Is it not time for the health care system to address funding treatment of patients here in Canada? The current population of patients is effectively untreated, or at the very least undertreated, and time continues to pass with their lives and health being compromised to what can only be considered an unacceptable extent.

The endless frustration of non-treatment (in other words, worsening of the symptoms of lymphedema) along with dealing with a medical community with little knowledge about lymphedema has a huge impact on patients, both physically and emotionally. At least more and more patients are informed of the risk of lymphedema before lymphadenectomy (lymph node removal) or radiation. I would have made different choices with regard to certain activities if I had known I was at risk for lymphedema post-surgically. These so-called 'routine procedures' have a dramatic impact on lives of many patients. Is any of this acceptable in a country that prides itself on its health care system?

Back to the personal, to be very honest there are times when I am quite down. For example when I go into a shoe store or shop for a bathing suit or lingerie. Or when I see someone jogging along the roadside, having what appears to be a fabulous run—I have to confess to a little jealousy when I remember how enjoyable running can be. Altogether, at times it is difficult not to resent the costs of having lymphedema—both financial and in terms of the time lymphedema consumes—as well as in terms of loss, that is the loss of opportunity to pursue those once-upon-a-time hobbies and physical activities that are now definitely out of the question. Having lymphedema forces you to dream up some different opportunities and lymphedema-appropriate physical activities.

In an image-conscious society, it is impossible to ignore the so-called 'vanity' aspect of lymphedema. Every morning, after my shower, in which the water must be on the cool side, and which nonetheless makes my legs feel even heavier and hotter after standing while bathing and washing my hair, I sit on my bed with my legs extended before me and cream my legs and feet with Eucerin lotion. I bandage my toes, and wearing the 'charming' somehow out-of-context (in my bedroom) pink rubber gloves that help me tug, grip, and smooth the heavy material, I struggle into my Class 4 compression stockings, and so-called 'panty' that is more like the tightest rubber underwear/bike shorts you ever saw.

During that time, it is difficult not to reflect on lymphedema and how it makes me feel: extremely unattractive, absolutely un-sexy, and bulge-y. I remember my legs and lingerie and hosiery and shoes of the days before lymphedema became a part of my life. How could I have been so reckless as to have taken my pre-cancer, pre-lymphedema, body for granted?

Every day, to put it mildly, I feel rather sad while I get dressed—it is difficult not to, when I look at the state of my body, let alone the choices I am forced to make with regard to what I wear. What I would like to convey to you is this, "*It has been of real significance for me to give myself permission to have that sadness.*" To say, "*Well, I am sad about having this condition.*"

Rather than gloss over it, experiencing sadness is a perfectly legitimate response to lymphedema. By the time I have all of my 'gear' on and have put the ugly gloves out of sight in my bedside table, I am ready for the day and have begun to focus more on what I need to accomplish on that given day. I think that by giving myself permission to have those few moments of private sadness I can then move on to what is for me, typically, a productive day.

At night, I sleep in Reid Sleeves. As you likely know, they are bulky, Velcro-strapped gear, one per leg, toes to top-of-leg. Their effectiveness is based on the internal egg-carton shaped foam rubber, which presses a more or less grid pattern into the leg, helping alleviate surface fibrosis or hardening of lymph. While unattractive and rather warm, they are far easier to manage than the regimen of nightly compression bandaging I would otherwise have to follow, and I am grateful to have them.

When all is said and done, what are a few of the things I have learned (so far) from the challenges presented by having lymphedema?

I have learned that while helping others during my involvement in the LAO I also, if inadvertently, helped myself. Being involved made it necessary for me to understand lymphedema in greater depth, and I was able to take much comfort in knowing that I am not alone.

I wish I could state unequivocally that I have reconciled myself to lymphedema and its implications for my life, and the life of my family, but unfortunately that is not the case. It is still difficult, although I continue to work at it.

I try to make every effort to put on a brave face, in spite of an ongoing inner struggle. For me, the worst part is the changeability of my condition and my fear of what might lie ahead. Granted, nobody knows what might lie ahead, but I am beginning to realize that having lymphedema complicates just about everything.

I have also learned that even if your doctor doesn't yet know much about lymphedema, it is very important, for your own state of mind, that he or she be supportive. The doctor I have now, whom I first met in the emergency department during my first cellulitis infection, acknowledges that I know more about this condition than he does.

When I ask him for something with regard to caring for my lymphedema, he demonstrates his belief in me by responding positively. When I was trying to obtain a pair of Reid Sleeves, he admitted that he had never heard of them, but he asked me to tell him about them and then simply wrote the prescription. His support is tremendously important to me, especially after it was so difficult to get doctors to listen to me when my lymphedema was in its early stages.

I've learned that I have to be an educator about lymphedema—with my doctors, family and friends.

Having lymphedema also places you in the position of needing to learn how to say "no." There are times when you simply cannot participate in certain events or activities. You have to learn to state your needs or limitations.

I find I feel very awkward when people say, *"Oh, you STILL have that? I thought you went for treatment."* All that said, I refuse to allow lymphedema to be a central feature of our lives and try to maintain a 'culture of wellness' in our home.

Some of the physical things I have learned about coping are:

- Exercise. Exercise. Exercise. But gently. Gradually build up strength and endurance.

- Eat salty things only in the most minute quantities. This includes dill pickles, anchovies, cheese, many types of crackers, many if not most prepared foods (many of which contain a salt mine worth of sodium), including salad dressings.

- If you have to sit for a long time, get up and walk around as often as you can. Whenever possible, take the aisle seat.

- Drink lots and lots of water. Eventually, you will know where all the washrooms are.

- Pace yourself. Being prone to infections, I try not to 'over do it' but it is a difficult lesson to learn. I now know when I have an infection that my body has been trying to tell me, *"You are asking too much of me."* And that always comes as a real surprise because I still like to think I have the endurance to do *almost* anything.

- Carry a prescription for antibiotics at all times, and if you are going to be out of the country, have it filled before you go.

- Get regular MLD (manual lymph drainage). The Wittlinger Clinic in Austria recommends one hour per week, which may not be affordable or even possible. But any MLD is better than none.

One doctor who specializes in lymphedema has told me I need to diminish the amount of stress in my life. Trying to appraise the stress in my life, my first thought was, *"The most stressful thing in my life is having lymphedema."*

Perhaps a condition with so many variables can't help but be stressful, as I feel I am always second-guessing the reasons for symptoms being better or worse, and trying to adapt.

All of these aspects are ultimately about being more self-aware and in control of your environment than you might have to be otherwise. As well, while many of the requirements for coping with lymphedema are time-consuming and dully repetitive, they have to become part of your daily life or your lymphedema will be placed at risk for worsening.

In closing, what I have related to you is only a blurry snapshot from my journey so far. Like everyone else's, my journey has been up and down, sometimes zigzagging sideways. Many of the features of my journey are things we, as lymphedema patients, have in common: the lack of information, sometimes wrong information, and frustration with the options or utter lack of options presented to us.

Sometimes though, we have been lucky and met excellent guides. Something else that we have in common is that we have all suffered a loss – the loss of the state of healthiness we experienced before, and all that is encompassed by that, and we have experienced what must be described as a compromised recovery. There has been a cost to our recovery from cancer, which we continue to pay, on a daily basis.

With regard to patients who suffer from lymphedema from causes other than cancer, and primary lymphedema patients, I feel that ultimately it doesn't matter how you got it—lymphedema is lymphedema, and it presents many identical life-long challenges to us all.

Like we all do, to the best of our ability, I continue to strive to meet those challenges with as much insight, humor (sometimes the most difficult) and grace (also quite difficult at times) as I can find within myself.

Joanne Young

My Son Is a Pretty Average Kid

"It is hard to wear long pants when you live in the South and its hot most of the year!"

Editors' Note: It can be pretty scary when your infant's legs start to swell and your doctor can't tell you what's wrong or what to do. 'Mom' shares her perspective as her son is growing up.

Jonathan is now 10 and he is a pretty average kid—except that he has primary lymphedema. I read stories about how other people grew up not having friends because of this disease and it breaks my heart. Happily, Jonathan has been accepted by his classmates.

They all know he wears a stocking on his leg and occasionally comes to school with bandages under his pants and that he gets to ride the elevator instead of climbing the stairs at school—and they think that is cool too.

As Jonathan has been growing up, we've helped him to gain independence and acceptance in learning to live well with his lymphedema. It doesn't slow him down, his classmates accept him, and he doesn't worry a lot about it.

His only complaint is that it is hard to wear long pants when you live in the South where it is hot most of the year!

Mom

I've Had Lymphedema for 71 Years

"I am so thankful that lymphedema information is finally coming out!"

Editors' Note: A Lymph Notes member graciously shares her story of living with lymphedema for 71 years!

I was born in 1926 and had erysipelas several times before the age of six. (As you may know, erysipelas is a form cellulitis in which the skin is bright red and noticeably swollen. Having lymphedema puts you at risk for erysipelas.)

At age 10 I had a very high fever and pneumonia. This happened before either sulfa drugs or penicillin. My doctor treated me with a mustard plaster and an oxygen tent.

After this illness, I had an unexplained swelling in my right ankle. Ten years later, at age 20, the swelling spread to my left ankle and leg.

I am now 81 years of age and have lived with lymphedema for 71 years.

Oklahoma is still one of the few states with very few treatment centers. My doctors here still have little or no knowledge of the condition.

I am so thankful that lymphedema information is finally coming out.

Lymph Notes Member

I Count My Blessings Every Day

" I believe you can learn to live with lymphedema and still have a good life."

Editors' Note: Betty's story makes us grateful both for the progress that has been made in treatment and for the fact that it is easier to learn about lymphedema and its treatment today. We hope that Betty's story, and all the stories in this book, spread the word that "you can learn to live with lymphedema and to still have a good life" and that lymphedema deserves more attention with better treatments and adequate insurance coverage for treatment.

My name is Betty and I'm sharing my story in the hope that others can learn from it. I was born 73 years ago with swelling of my left foot, leg, and part of the left side of my body. I have learned that this is congenital primary lymphedema. In all of my years, I have never met anyone else with this condition.

As a child, my Mother took me to many clinics but no one could provide any help. When I was 12 we went to the Mayo Clinic. All they could offer me was to wrap my leg with large heavy rubber bandages.

When I was 15 we heard of a clinic in Texas where a doctor was working with lymph patients. When we went to him my leg and foot were huge with swelling. I had four operations on my leg in which tissue was removed from below my knee to my ankle and some from my foot. I also had many skin grafts. That was the last time I was professionally treated for this condition.

As a child I swam, biked, ice skated, ran, and played baseball. As an adult I worked as a cashier, married, had two sons, and was always active. I'm still active and have pretty normal life.

I wish lymphedema were not such a "hidden disease". I'm happy that it is beginning to get more attention with better treatments available. I believe you can learn to live with lymphedema and to still have a good life. Therefore, despite having been through some the hard times, I count my blessings every day.

Betty

I am the Queen of Lymphedema

"I have a great outlook on life and I am forever grateful to be here."

Editors' Note: Lymphedema can make you self-conscious or fearful of how others will react. Here is a wonderful example of a woman who has had lymphedema for 47 years and hasn't let it stop her.

Hi! My name is Shirley Glick and I celebrated my 75th birthday on May 24, 2007. I had radical breast surgery when I was 28 years old. This makes it more than 47 years that I have been living with lymphedema!! This is why I jokingly refer to myself as *"The Queen of Lymphedema."* I would love to contribute to this book.

I worked as a high school home economics teacher. At that time knit compression sleeves, which can be hidden under a blouse, were not being used. This made it more difficult to work with high school students, given their mentality toward something different. However, I successfully made it to retirement. Since retiring, I have had my own antique business for the past 15 years and that keeps me occupied.

Oh yes, and did I mentioned that I was divorced? The experience of reentering the "dating world" with one breast and lymphedema was a challenging one! But I overcame it.

While I was writing, my marvelous lymphatic drainage massage therapist, Joan Glunk (see page 53), called to wish me luck. She has been doing massage on me for the past nine years and is a true inspiration!!!!

Despite all of my experiences with lymphedema, I have a great outlook on life and I am forever grateful to be here so I could savor the experiences I have been given in life. Seventy five years is pretty good odds and I am happy to have had them!

Shirley Glick

I Have Learned So Much from My Therapist

"It amazes me that there is so little knowledge in the general public about this condition."

Editors' Note: CM shares the first steps of her journey of learning to live well with lymphedema.

Where are you in your journey? We offer these stories so the "voices" of others will be your companions on this journey offering support, encouragement, and guidance.

I had surgery for breast cancer on August 29, 2006. They took out five lymph nodes. My upper arm was swollen afterwards and numb on the backside, but my surgeon said it might, or might not, go away.

I wasn't too worried about it. At my last checkup he said he was 90% sure I'd never get lymphedema.

All I knew about lymphedema was what I'd read in a Cancer Society booklet. It said I didn't want to get it, and to not let anyone take my blood pressure or blood in that arm. That was all I knew!

During radiation, I developed a bad burn under my arm above where the lymph nodes were taken out. It opened up and when it healed, it caused scar tissue. About a month before my treatments ended, my hand began to swell.

I didn't realize what it was, so it was two weeks before I mentioned it to the doctor. She said it could be a blood clot in my arm or lymphedema and to keep an eye on it. She never asked about it again so I didn't worry much about it.

When I went to the next cancer doctor, she sent me immediately to get fitted for a sleeve. I left for a week's vacation and wore the sleeve for a few days but realized it was making my hand swell more so I took it off and left it off until I started therapy the next week.

The therapist wrapped my hand from the knuckles up to my underarm. That caused my fingers to swell. From then on she wrapped them from the fingertips.

My insurance allowed me to go twice a week for four weeks of massage therapy. At the end, I was given a prescription for a glove that would cost $225.

I didn't order the custom-made glove because the insurance wouldn't pay for it. Instead I bought an off-the-shelf glove that fits either hand but has uncomfortable ridges in the fingers. It was still $156. Now I'm thinking about going back and ordering the other one for $225 hoping it will be more comfortable to wear.

I learned from my therapist that I have to be careful of infections, cuts, manicures, the sun, hot water, and bug bites. Shortly after being wrapped near the end of my therapy, I fell on that arm and skinned my hand right through all the bandages. I now have an antibiotic prescription from my doctor with no date on it, in case I do get an infection and I can't get to him right away.

It amazes me that there is so little knowledge in the general public about this condition. When people ask me what's wrong with my arm because of the sleeve and glove, they have no idea what I'm talking about when I tell them. Even friends and family who are learning with me don't really under-stand.

I don't remember how I found out about the Lymph Notes forum (www.lymphnotes.com), but it's been a real help to me as I learn more and it gives me the opportunity to ask questions and get answers from people who understand and are going through the same thing.

I just had my check-up with my radiation doctor and told her I thought the lymphedema was caused by the radiation, but she didn't want to accept that. I just picked up the book **Living Well With Lymphedema** today and can't wait to read it and learn more about how to help myself live well.

Editors' Note: CM's story continues, read on to find out what happens.

Since my diagnosis with secondary lymphedema I've been working with my therapist to get a compression glove that would fit properly. Finally we had to order a custom glove from Germany.

While waiting for it to arrive, I got a small bug bite on my affected arm. I didn't do anything about it and after several weeks the redness and itching finally went away; however the increased swelling did not retreat.

My custom glove finally arrived; however as soon as I put it on, I knew it wasn't right. The fingers were too small and tight. Despite the discomfort I wore it for several hours just to be sure. When I took it off there was a deep wound-like indentation and redness around the base of my thumb.

Since my oncologist was on maternity leave, I saw the doctor who was substituting for her. His first question when he saw my sleeve was, *"Aren't you getting into this sleeve thing a little early?"*

When I took the glove off to show him the wound he said, *"Oh, don't worry about that – but you really should lose some weight."* His final recommendation was, *"Just skip the glove and sleeve and be more comfortable."*

When I told him that would make the swelling worse his reaction was, *"So what as long as you can still function?"* He was not at all worried about infection and was convinced that my quality of life would be better if I were more comfortable without wearing all that compression stuff.

After reading the book **Living Well With Lymphedema,** I knew enough not to listen to him! When I saw my primary care physician the next day, I took the book with me.

This doctor admitted that, *"All they taught us in medical school was not to draw blood or take blood pressure on that arm and put a sleeve on it."* He then prescribed the antibiotics needed to treat the infection and wrote the prescription needed to continue with my lymphedema treatment.

CM

My Lymphedema Journey

"KEEP on keeping on!"

Editors' Note: Judy's story is another wonderful example of the importance of perseverance. We hope you enjoy sharing her journey.

Sixteen years ago, I underwent the removal of lymph nodes due to adeno-carcinoma of the cervix and uterus. Within two months of this surgery, I developed lymphedema in my left leg. The doctors were not familiar with lymphedema and the swelling caused alarm that it might be another tumor.

I endured a second surgery just seven months after the initial surgery. The second surgery resulted in increased swelling, more irritation, and escalated discomfort.

In order to receive the much-needed treatment for lymphedema, I had to travel over 90 miles from my home to San Francisco. For more than two years I made that long journey to and from San Francisco, where I would spend full days on the pump, and receive MLD treatments scattered throughout the day.

I would leave in full bandages, make the long journey back home, only to return the next day and do it all over again. At that time, San Francisco was the only available facility that offered MLD. In addition, my insurance did not recognize lymphedema as a disease, so my treatments were considered "an alternative treatment" that was not covered by my insurance.

A few years later, more people had learned about lymphedema so that both treatment and support groups were offered in San Jose. It was still 45 miles away from home, but a lot closer than the 90 miles I had been previously traveling to San Francisco.

When I began working at Santa Cruz Radiation Oncology, I was privileged to receive strong support from Dr. Mann and Dr. Sacks, who arranged a meeting with the Dominican Hospital Rehabilitation Facility Director, Dr. Quinn.

I was able to provide Dr. Quinn and his team with the codes and costs associated with lymphedema treatment, as well as the documentation necessary to show that MLD was a viable treatment that Dominican Hospital could offer. Dr. Quinn was extremely proactive and set up the Physical Therapy Department of Dominican Hospital with a lymphedema treatment program.

My initial treatment at Dominican Hospital was with Johanna, an RN who also has lymphedema. Johanna embraced the program and through her hard work and dedication she was able to get the program off the ground. After my initial experience, I am thrilled to see that Santa Cruz has a growing dynamic lymphedema program with a caring and creative therapist at the helm. Dominican Hospital now offers a caring touch for a very misunderstood condition that can be disabling, both physically and emotionally, to those who suffer with it.

It goes without saying that it is my deepest desire that a cure for lymphedema will soon be discovered. Until then, our doctors need to be informed of this condition and able to provide medical treatment and support.

To my fellow lymphedema patients I would like to say, "*KEEP on keeping on!*" I would also like to thank Dominican Hospital for their continued support and all of you who have worked so hard on our fundraisers. (For more information on these fundraisers see page 158.)

Judy Gloeckler

Facing Lymphedema

"It was only after several medical appointments that I heard the word lymphedema for the first time."

Editors' Note: Brent recounts his personal journey first to get a diagnosis and then to accept the diagnosis. In Activities (page 87) and Self-Care Tips (page 136), you will read more about how lymphedema has changed Brent's life – in some ways for the better!

My name is Brent. My coming to terms with the condition of lymphedema initially was complicated by my medical professionals' unfamiliarity with the condition. These doctors sent me in various unfruitful directions and it was only after several medical appointments that I heard the word lymphedema for the first time.

Then, unfortunately, a lymphedema diagnosis seemed to be assigned by default. That is, if no other condition could be determined, it must be lymphedema. This was not satisfying, and for a considerable period, I believed that someone must know more about what was affecting me than the medical professionals whom I was encountering.

I visited every type of alternative practitioner I could think of. Only when all options were exhausted did I acknowledge that perhaps this was incurable, was lymphedema, and was a genuine medical condition.

Discovering a book on the topic was of significant help in coming to recognize that I did indeed have lymphedema. Another step was acquiring information from fact sheets and websites.

Also of great help was talking with health care professionals whose practices center on lymphedema and who are more familiar with the condition than any of the doctors I had encountered.

Brent

Thankfulness Comes Easy

"When I start to feel sad about myself I remember all of my blessings. That helps me so much."

Editors' Note: This story captures how we not only want to notice what helps us physically, but what helps and supports us emotionally.

After radiation treatment for cervical cancer, I have lymphedema in both legs, some severe stomach problems etc. Every day, thanks to my husband, I get an MLD massage and he helps me with my compression hose (not too romantic). Every night I wrap. Sometimes I wrap during the day because of the pain.

Thankfulness comes easy in my family. They are all so supportive and helpful. We put our concerns on the important things in life: the babies. We have an abundant crop and we love every one of them.

There is a lot of healing in holding a new little person and feeding them. There is also a lot of joy in getting them that new little special thing they wanted or taking them to the planetarium.

When I start to feel sad about myself I remember all of my blessings: my children are healthy and working and all of my grandchildren are healthy and studying hard. That helps me so much.

Lymph Notes Member

I Live a Full and Very Active Life

"I have four children, worked full time as a nurse, have led a full life, and also have lymphedema."

Editors' Note: Bonnie's story reflects how difficult it can be to get a diagnosis and find treatment for primary lymphedema. One of the things we find so heartening is that she has a "full and very active life" with work, travel, and parenting despite lymphedema.

Among other things, her story illustrates the theme of doing what you can even if it's not 'perfect', and noticing what works so you can monitor your lymphedema and keep doing what keeps it controlled.

Hi my name is Bonnie Moats. My left leg starting swelling during my first pregnancy. The doctors were concerned and ordered for me to stay off it, wrap it with an Ace bandage, and lie down on the floor with my leg propped up against the wall.

With my second pregnancy, the swelling got worse so after delivery the doctor sent me to a specialist in varicose veins. He diagnosed me with primary lymphedema and told me it had no cause and no cure.

In 1977, thirty years ago, I was fitted with a Jobst stocking up to my knee for daytime use. Around 1990, a friend from work read an article in Parade magazine about lymphedema with a Dr. Lerner who had studied in Germany and had clinics in New York and New Jersey.

I called for an appointment and was scheduled for four weeks of massage therapy. Each week, Monday through Friday, I arrived for two treatments a day. They taught me how to bandage etc. This was all very new and it really helped me!

I am now 53 and have lived a full and very active life. I have four kids, three boys and one girl; plus I worked full time as a nurse. Between work and home I was on my feet all the time! The kids were involved in a lot so I didn't have time to sit with my legs up. I just used a CircAid stocking and wrappings at night.

I have flown overseas to visit my children and went with little sleep to watch my grandson. I work out with exercise equipment a lot and I have had no problems. In fact, last year the therapist said that my leg had gotten smaller.

There was never much information on lymphedema and most people never heard of it. Thanks to the Lord and the friend I had who found that clinic. I am glad that some information will be going out there for others.

Bonnie Moats

The Joy of Living

"Those of us dealing with this condition may not like the reality of lymphedema, but we can rise to meet the challenge."

Editors' Note: In this moving story, Mary opens her heart and welcomes us to join her on her journey through 'shock, dismay, and a chilling fear' back to laughter and joy. Come along for the ride!

It is hard to believe that twenty years have passed since I was given the diagnosis of malignant melanoma. The doctor's voice resonates in my memory and I can visualize myself in the sterile examining room of the Grace Hospital in St. John's, Newfoundland, Canada. As his voice drones on about the type of surgery needed for this condition, the green walls seem to move closer. Finally, he asks me how I feel about the coming ordeal. My only response is that I need to go home and prepare supper. Shock, dismay, and a chilling fear grip me on the drive home as I absorb the implications.

Two days later I received life-saving and life-altering surgery on my left leg. I require painful skin grafts and the removal of lymph nodes. All surgery is serious but this becomes worse than I thought. I had a catheter in my spine for morphine to control the pain.

However, one incident stands out in memory which shows us how the human spirit can be helped by humor. One day, through a haze of morphine, I look up to see seven handsome young male medical students enter my room and encircle my hospital bed. Apparently, they find my surgery very interesting. As I lay there, more or less exposed in an ill-fitting Johnny coat, I hear *"Amazing!"*, *"How interesting!"*, *"Look at that!"*, *"I am glad to have the opportunity to see this!"* The situation suddenly becomes funny to me and I can't help but laugh. After an awkward moment, the students look at each other and we all laugh together, even my rather serious surgeon.

Difficult days lay ahead. I am informed that as a result of the surgery, I can expect some permanent swelling in my leg. At the time, however, it seems the lesser of two evils: one, I can die; or two, I can live with swelling in my leg. Right then and there I became thankful not to be relegated to the first choice. The seriousness of my condition reveals itself over the next few months.

I believe I have coped with the swelling, or the lymphedema, because of the forward thinking of my surgeon. He explains to me that I will need to wear a compression garment to keep the swelling under control. He even has me measured for a custom stocking before being discharged. While I am waiting for the stocking, a nurse shows me how to wrap bands of cloth around my leg. The doctor goes on to explain the importance of cleanliness and avoiding infection. He suggests that for thirty minutes a day, I lie on the floor with my leg straight up on the wall to allow the fluid to drain, and he tells me to go for long brisk walks.

Perhaps the most important thing he says to me, in a gentle but firm voice, is to comply with his instructions or expect serious complications. I remember his words, his expression, and his concern for me. I am forever thankful for the time he has taken to prepare me for a lifetime of dealing with lymphedema.

The physical dimensions of this condition are serious enough, but the psychological impact presents its own challenges. At age thirty-eight, a junior high school teacher with active teenagers at home, I felt I had the world by the tail. Believing myself to be fairly attractive and successful, I had a healthy self-esteem.

Suddenly I became conscious of an ugly surgical stocking with a wide seam up the back as the most obvious part of my wardrobe. This I must wear all day, every day. It never seemed to look right with my clothes. My lovely dresses and skirts hung in the closet and I began to replace them with trousers. Shorts and swimsuits were out of the question. The pain of surgery pales in comparison to the attack on my vanity.

How easy it is to feel sorry for yourself! I must admit to wallowing in self-pity for a while. Slowly, I began to see the light, and although I do not claim to be wise in many things, I believe I have achieved some enlightenment.

I allow myself to be carried along by the everyday necessities, dealing with work, family responsibilities, and church. It has been my great fortune to see my children finish school and university. We have traveled together and my husband and I have enjoyed their achievements. Going for long walks with my cherished boarder collie, Rosie, is a source of great joy.

I am especially thankful that I can sing in choirs and participate in all the activities I love and recently my husband and I have taken up ballroom dancing. I also continued my teaching career right up to retirement.

Twenty years after surgery, lymphedema has become part of my routine, part of my life. The key word is "part". It has not taken over nor restricted me. I continue to be informed and do the necessary things to lessen the impact of this condition. Presently, I am receiving therapy from a nurse who specializes in lymphedema treatments. That is not to say that there are no longer moments, when on a trip or cruise, I wish that stocking did not exist.

The French use an expression "*Joie de Vivre*," joy of living. I think that is the secret to adapting to change and embracing new realities. Those of us dealing with this condition may not like the reality of lymphedema, but we can rise to meet the challenge.

Mary D. Warren

I Am No Longer Super Woman

"I have been given a gift of life and I want to share."

Editors' Note: Martha speaks of how she "looks for the learning experience that comes from life changes." She has responded to cancer and lymphedema by affirming through painting and by courageously learning to ask for and accept help.

I stare at my hand and my arm noting the size, the puffy fat skin.

Yesterday I was Super Woman. Doing, doing, doing, never any concern for me. Why should I? It has been six years without incident since my breast cancer. This couldn't happen to me – I am Super Woman! Well, no longer. I sit with tears in my eyes. Knowing I have to get help but being unable to think, all I can do is sit and cry.

I remember how I reached out for help when I found out that I had breast cancer. By taking things into my own hands, with the support of my close family, I made decisions and took action. These were changes I didn't ask for, but challenges that were given to me.

In looking for the learning experience that comes from life changes, I discovered that I must create. Painting became my outlet, to let everyone see the beauty of our world through my eyes. I had been given a gift of life and I want to share those feelings with others through my paintings.

Now I have another challenge presented to me: lymphedema of my hand and arm. This is a big reminder that I am *not* Super Woman. I need to work with others to get tasks done. I just can't do it all by myself anymore. There are a lot of people out there who want to help me, but don't know what I need done. I need to swallow my pride and ask. This is a hard lesson for me to learn, but slowly I ask for help.

Now I seek the learning experience that is to come from this life change. The garments that control my swelling are not beautiful (but they do work). I need to find something that will help me feel beautiful, inside and out. I still want to celebrate my femininity, to let my inner beauty show, and to let that beauty radiate out.

Martha Ruppert

I Remember Those Feelings

"Lymphedema is not my life anymore"

Editors' Note: Tracy tells of her journey through fear and depression to not feeling like a "victim of lymphedema".

I remember having such strong, fearful, and depressing emotions when I was first diagnosed. Now I'm so used to it and I find so many ways around this handicap called lymphedema, that it doesn't seem that big a deal anymore.

Not to make light of it, but lymphedema is not my life anymore, the way it was when I first developed it. I wonder, is this new, somewhat cavalier attitude, due to the fact that I live in a place where I get excellent care from wonderful lymphedema therapists and there is also a support group where I can share my fears and concerns and then let go of them?

I'm not scared any more because I know there are medical professionals within a very short distance who can help me when I have trouble. They've been doing it for years! Not to mention the wonderful books and websites like Lymph Notes. Knowledge is power and I don't feel the victim of lymphedema anymore. I do what I'm supposed to do to manage it. Exercise, diet, compression garments, night sleeves, massage, etc. I manage it, it doesn't manage me!

But I do feel extremely lucky that there is help where I live. And that I have health insurance. I know that many, many people do not have the care and options that I have available to me. I do not take these things for granted and I count my blessings every day. I pray for the day where everyone who needs it, will get the lymphedema care they require.

Tracy Novak

My World Improved in Leaps and Bounds

"My life has returned to a very active one and is beautiful."

Editors' Note: This moving story from a Lymph Notes member tells a journey from being told he was going to die to surviving and living a rich, full life now 16 years later. He is now an active grandfather and a school bus driver.

Having been diagnosed with primary lymphedema in 1989, I had already spent two years during which doctors were confused, concerned, and really did not know which way to turn. In hospital one midnight I had been told that I would not be alive the following morning and that I should make peace with God and my family. It was very scary and sobering to say the least!

Three specialists were present: one in internal medicine, one in infectious diseases, and the third a skin doctor. As the swelling was manifested in both legs, they tried inflatable pressure on both legs and feet. This provided only very temporary relief.

After one of them learned of a physiotherapist who had recently returned to Canada from the United States where she had studied the treatment of lymphedema through gentle pressure and two-way stretch bandages, my world improved in leaps and bounds. My weight went down by over fifty pounds in my legs alone.

Now, 16 years later, I still take low dosage penicillin twice daily and wear compression stockings reverting to bandages every two or three weeks for one day. Life has returned to a very active one and is beautiful. I have now been married to the same beautiful lady for 45 years and we have 11 grandchildren.

Lymph Notes Member

I Am a Therapeutic Clown

"Humor is important to getting well."

Editors' Note: Marty's story is an unusual one. We had never heard of a 'therapeutic clown' before she contacted us, and we think it's a great idea.

I am a therapeutic clown. You would be surprised, but there are a lot of us around. We go into the hospitals, nursing homes, assisted living facilities, and my favorite: cancer centers.

I have been a professional clown for over 20 years, but it wasn't until I was diagnosed with breast cancer that I realized how important humor is to getting well.

I have not let lymphedema stop me from clowning and, dressed as my clown character, compression garments don't show. I have been attending classes and different courses over the last five years in the USA and Canada so that now I am a certified therapeutic clown.

It cracks me up when people ask me what I do for living and I tell them. They think I am joking but I'm not. You should see me!

Marty

Editors' Note: If you are interested in learning about therapeutic clowning, start by looking at these websites:

www.caringclownsinternational.org, www.caringclowns.org, www.therapeuticclownscanada.ca, and www.hospitalclowns.org.

Chapter **2**

Stories from Professionals

Editors' Note: The best lymphedema therapists bring head, hands, and heart to their work. The first four stories reflect how patients serve as inspiration to the professionals who treat them. In the final three stories of this chapter therapists share the journeys that led them to this profession and how they think about their work.

My Patients Are Truly Inspiring

Editors' Note: This remark by Joan Glunk who is a licensed massage therapist (LMT) and a certified lymphedema therapist (CLT) summed up the beautiful way that someone with lymphedema can be a source of inspiration to others.

My patients are truly inspiring and have a wealth of knowledge not only about caring for their limbs but living robustly despite their lymphedema. They surprise and humble me on a daily basis.

Joan Glunk, LMT, CLT

AZ Goes to Wal-Mart

"When I first met him, AZ was 57 and had been bedridden for about 30 years"

Editors' Note: Untreated lymphedema can be painful and disabling. In this wonderful story James Morrow and his colleagues help a bedridden patient lose several hundred pounds of swelling and regain his mobility.

I have been a therapist about seven years now and patients are always inspiring me. One who is especially significant to me is AZ.

When I first met him, AZ was 57 and had been bedridden for about 30 years. Both legs and feet were huge. It was estimated that his right leg alone weighed between 300 and 400 pounds. The swelling was from the knees down. In all other areas, he was a normal size with some abdominal swelling. When he would try to stand, the weight would pull down so hard that blood vessels would break and he would be in severe pain for several days.

It was impossible to reach around the leg to apply the bandages so it took two therapists, working together as a team, to treat and bandage his legs. The first thing we did was to massage him and then wrap the legs. I then pulled the weight up with bandages and attached this to the thighs being careful not to restrict the fluid. This allowed him to stand without having the weight break the blood vessels behind the knee.

I then asked him to get out of bed each day and touch the wall. With treatment and movement the fluid began to reduce and finally we could apply the bandages with only one person. His fluid seemed to stabilize so we began to use Komprex Binde (padding) stretched tightly under the bandage. Again the fluid reduced. When it stabilized again, I decided to use Komprex foam chips. His legs were so fibrotic that the chips barely dented them. I thought I would make bigger chips so I would roll Komprex Binde into rolls about 1 to 2 inch diameter and place these under the Komprex Binde that was rolled on. The tissue would soften and then reduce.

He was now walking more. He went to the kitchen and back, then around the house, then to the street and then to the end of the block. After a year he and his wife were walking on the beach most afternoons. He reported they would usually walk between one half to one mile. He was now small enough that his wife could bandage him.

In the beginning it took 75 bandages to cover one of AZ's legs from the foot to the knee. His wife would wash and have these rolled for every visit. He never complained and did everything he was asked to do without complaint. My biggest problem was slowing him down so he would not overtire the leg.

On his first day of treatment, I asked him what he wanted to accomplish and he said he would like to see what was inside a Wal-Mart since he had never been to a big store like that. Now, I hate going to Wal-Mart and always used to complain about standing in line for such a long time to check-out. AZ achieved his goal. He went to Wal-Mart and had a ball—and I've stopped complaining about shopping or standing in line.

Thanks to AZ, many people around here have a whole new look at a lot of things.

James Morrow, MT, CLT-LANA

Enabling My Patient to Feel Well

"This story demonstrates how lymphedema can hold a victim hostage for years if proper treatment is not available."

Editors' Note: Paula Stewart, MD, CLT-LANA is a caring physician and a marvelous speaker. She shares this encouraging story "to demonstrate that treatment is available and can change lives impacted by lymphedema regardless of the cause."

This story is about my first lymphedema patient as a staff physician in Charlotte, North Carolina. My teacher and mentor at the Mayo Clinic called me shortly after my arrival to ask if I would see and treat Frances, a patient who had traveled to Mayo for treatment of longstanding lymphedema and who lived near Charlotte. Arrangements were made for Frances to be seen in our clinic within days of her return home.

In the few months that I had been working in the area, I had established a Cancer Rehab team and had found dedicated outpatient therapists to see and treat lymphedema patients. We felt ready to provide treatment, but Frances was a bit doubtful that we could help her. She had seen many doctors over the 20 years that she had been plagued with lymphedema.

The lymphedema had developed days after her modified radical mastectomy for breast cancer. She had had over 30 lymph nodes removed in a level two lymphadenectomy for staging.

Within days of her surgery Frances was sick with a wound infection. In addition to the pain and fever, she had swelling and went on to develop cellulitis, an infection of the subcutaneous tissues in the affected arm. She was treated with broad-spectrum antibiotics and was discharged home.

The swelling did not resolve and approximately three months later she had another bout of cellulitis. She was treated with oral antibiotics again with complete resolution of her symptoms, except for the swelling in her right arm, which was slowly worsening with time. It was not getting better as her surgeon had predicted.

Over the next 20 years, Frances suffered from repeated bouts of cellulitis approximately every three to four months. Most of these episodes included severe malaise for a day or two followed by intense redness and warmth and pain of her left arm. Sometimes she suffered a high fever.

Most of the time she was treated with oral antibiotics at home, but on seven occasions she was hospitalized and during five of those hospitalizations she required intubation and ventilator support due to sepsis and respiratory failure. And with each episode her arm was a little larger. Over time her infections were worse.

Frances was tired of her illness and pain and especially unhappy that her arm was so large it no longer fit into her clothing. She was grateful that the doctors had saved her life so many times but she wanted someone to stop the repeated infections and the swelling in her arm.

On evaluation, Frances' left arm was visibly larger than her right and measured about 7 centimeters (2.8 inches) larger in circumference on average. The skin was fibrotic (hardened) and somewhat discolored. It felt heavy to her and she had occasional shooting pains in her forearm. Her mastectomy scar was well healed and there were no signs of infection in her arm. There were no swollen lymph nodes in her neck or axilla (armpit).

She was scheduled for three weeks of outpatient therapy, three times a week. She was very compliant with the program and treatment. At the end of the program, her arm measured only 2 cm (0.8 inches) larger than the unaffected arm.

This was a thrilling moment for her. Finally, her arm was small enough to fit into her clothing again! She was fitted with a custom made one-piece compressive sleeve with glove and which she wore from awakening to bedtime every day.

I followed Frances as an outpatient for 10 years and in that time she suffered only one bout of cellulitis after she absentmindedly bit a hangnail from her affected limb thumb. She called immediately with the first signs of infection and we successfully treated the cellulitis with a round of oral antibiotics.

Frances continued to wear her garment every day over the years and, with time, her affected arm measured almost the same as her unaffected arm. She was so grateful to be free of the chronic infections and illness that she became a fan of the program and our lymphedema treatment. She often came to lectures I gave in the region, discussed her experiences and success with treatment, and modeled her slim, infection-free arm.

Her story demonstrates how lymphedema can hold a victim hostage for years if proper treatment is not available. For 20 years Frances felt ill more often than well because of the recurrent cellulitis that was associated with her untreated lymphedema.

With standard treatment and simple daily maintenance, Frances was able to feel well, wear her beloved wardrobe, and be free of pain and illness.

Paula Stewart, MD, CLT-LANA

Betty's Journey Toward Healing

"Courage, strength, and determination..."

Editors' Note: Liz Pomeroy shares her story about an inspiring patient. Think about the ways in which you may be an inspiration to others in your life as well. For every one person who has been publicly honored, we believe there are hundreds of others who deserve it. We nominate YOU, Dear Reader.

The management of lymphedema requires a lifetime commitment and one person who has made this commitment is Betty Oertel. Betty is an elementary school music teacher with a severe form of primary lymphedema known as lipo-lymphedema which is a combination of lipedema and lymphedema.

About 10 or 15 years ago, Betty spent four hours a day on a form of pump treatment that we no longer prescribe in an attempt to rid her body of excess fluid. When this did not work Betty was convinced that she was "just fat," so she set out to lose weight on a medically-supervised liquid diet. She reports, *"I lost 70 pounds, but my legs kept growing."*

About a year-and-a-half ago, doctors began talking about amputating her left leg. "At that time, they were estimating that my left leg alone weighed 100 pounds," Betty said. Instead she was referred to our clinic for MLD treatment.

Before she started treatment, Betty could not get into bed without help from her husband, she couldn't sit in a recliner, and she had extreme difficulty getting into and out of a car. Now a smiling Betty reports, *"I actually can see my ankle, which I had not seen in years. Also I can get into bed on my own, can rollover by myself, and get in and out of cars much more easily."*

Initially, Betty received therapy five times a week. The number of visits per week has gradually been reduced and our goal is to have Betty maintain her gains through self-care at home.

Betty's self-care program includes daily exercises, deep abdominal breathing, self-massage to help reroute the lymph, and plenty of water consumption. Exercise and getting the joints and limbs to move is important, you have to use your muscle pumps to help push out the fluid. Deep breathing is important because the majority of lymph nodes are in the abdomen and neck.

The staff at the Fort HealthCare Therapy and Lymphedema Center honored Betty by nominating her for a NLN 2007 Lymphedema Awareness "D" Day award *for her courage, strength, and determination in dealing with lymphedema.*

Betty Oertel is a charismatic, determined woman who has been fighting bilateral lower extremity lymphedema courageously for half her life. She has fought with a positive attitude through the treatment process and has come a long way to improve her independence and self confidence. Betty is a queen among patients and an inspiration to all who meet her.

Liz Pomeroy, OTR, CLT-LANA

Why I became a Lymphedema Therapist

"Once I started the training courses I knew I was, finally, in the right role."

Editors' Note: Doris Laing shares her journey to becoming a lymphedema therapist. Doris' story provides insight into the training required. To learn more about who is trained in effective lymphedema treatment, see Diagnosis and Treatment (page 70).

After working in a Physical Therapy Department as an office manager, I realized that I wanted to become a physical therapist; however, sometimes life requires some fancy footwork to reach your goal. As a single Mom, I knew I'd have to combine working with school. Therefore my first stop was our local State University to take prerequisite courses to enable me to apply to physical therapy (PT) school. At the same, time I worked as a waitress for a local Italian restaurant.

Unfortunately, me and a thousand other physical-therapist want-to-be's, were in the same boat and there weren't enough openings to transfer into a local PT program. As a staff member of the PT department, I was able to work in a clinical setting and I got to interact with patients as I managed appointment scheduling and related responsibilities. I had not given up my dream and at night I took advanced anatomy, physiology, and related courses.

I stayed with my original job and one day the physical therapist asked me to schedule a massage appointment outside the clinic for one of our patients. Only one problem, our hospital didn't have a massage therapist. As office manager, my job was to bring revenue in, not refer it out. Since I wanted to provide patient care, why not provide massage services to physical therapy patients? With encouragement and support from the department head and other staff therapists, I submitted a proposal to Human Resources to allow me to attend Massage Therapy School and return to treat patients as a licensed massage therapist.

To my delight, the proposal was approved. The only thing missing was finding a nearby school (this was before the Internet).

While pondering the school problem I happened to see a massage therapist friend on the street. We talked, he encouraged me to "go for it" and he provided the necessary information. The program was six months in length and, in order to be away from the department for that long, I had to use up all of my vacation time, sick leave, personal days, and holidays. (Oh yes, I was still working that restaurant job on weekends and some evenings I even worked my old job at the hospital.)

After I became a licensed massage therapist, I returned to the physical therapy department and was happily part of the patient care team.

One day we got a phone call from a Physician's Assistant working in the hospital. She had lymphedema, her arm was swelling, and she needed help but she was hours away from her lymphedema therapist. Her arm needed to be bandaged and surely someone in the Physical Therapy department could help her. As the team was working on figuring out how to get her arm bandaged, the head of Physical Therapy happened to walk into the area. Her logical question was, *"Why aren't we providing this service? What kind of training does it require?"*

I contacted the patient's therapist and discovered that as a licensed massage therapist, I was eligible to train as a lymphedema therapist by taking a series of one-week courses. She explained that the National Lymphedema Network required at least 135 hours of post-graduate training for these therapists (based on LANA standards). Because I had not taken the same college level courses that physical therapists and occupational therapists had, I elected to enroll in the longer 160 hour training program offered by the Vodder School.

Once I started the Vodder courses I knew I was, finally, in the right role. I loved the work, the patients, and the feeling of service that it gave me. I completed my training and established the lymphedema treatment program in our hospital. It was very successful, and yet I wanted to prove to myself that it was "real" and that I was as well qualified as other therapists across the country. In order to prove this to myself, I took and passed the LANA certification examination. I have since relocated to another state and I know the LANA certification was instrumental in providing credibility to my knowledge and skills as a lymphedema therapist.

Today I continue to be enthusiastic about working as a lymphedema therapist. I enjoy going into work in the morning knowing that each patient will bring a special opportunity to do the work I love.

Recently I ran across a poem by Amy Hayes (on page 62) that touched me deeply and expresses how I feel that I have truly been blessed to be able to help and heal with God's love.

Doris Laing, LMT, CLT-LANA

"The Gift" by Amy Hayes

The Lord, He gave me these useful hands to do good deeds on earth.
Though until now I've been unsure just what these hands are worth.
Now I know without a doubt these hands were made to heal.
To think he gave me such a gift, a blessing so surreal.
So I will use them the best I can with compassion, tenderness and love.
And never let a day go by without thanking God above.
Should I ever be boastful of my gift and lose sign of his plan.
May I always be reminded -- It is HE that does the Healing,
I am just the hands.

From Small to Big

"I am glad that in this big country I can be of help."

Editors' Note: Dutch-born Alma Vinje-Harrewijn is our co-author for Living Well With Lymphedema. *Here she speaks in a very personal way of how her childhood experiences in the Netherlands help her understand what happens in manual lymph drainage.*

You may find yourself thinking of your lymph vessels in a whole new way after following Alma on her travels from "a small country to this big country of America".

This is my story of how I came to treat lymphedema, how I came from a small country to this big country of America, and how I think about lymphatic drainage. I hope my story underlines how important manual lymph drainage is as part of comprehensive decongestive therapy and that it helps you to appreciate the efforts certified lymphedema therapists make to maintain and improve lymphatic skills.

As you may be able to tell from my name, Alma Vinjé-Harrewijn, I am Dutch. I spent my childhood in a small dairy town in the Netherlands, near the North Sea. The Netherlands depends on a system of trenches, canals, sluices, and levees to channel away water that would otherwise flood the land.

As a young girl, I often accompanied one of the farmers when he cleaned the streams, removing the build-up of mud and dead water plants. Sitting on his tractor, I could see that once a creek was freed from debris, the water drained more easily.

Studying manual lymphatic drainage as a physical therapy student, I recognized how similar the lymph system is to the Dutch river systems where I grew up. Both need means of filtering, cleaning, and draining fluid that will otherwise build up and cause harm.

As I practiced manual lymph drainage, I visualized the vessels as little canals being cleaned by the different strokes. I pictured fluids being drained out of the tissues and debris carried away with it.

I still remember the first patient who came to me for treatment of her lymphedema. I reviewed all my notes from the training I'd received, but quickly realized that the brief schooling I had was not enough.

I eagerly completed postgraduate training in comprehensive lymphedema therapy and joined the Dutch organization of lymphedema physical therapists that publishes "Oedeminus," their quarterly journal.

Moving from a busy, full-time practice in the Netherlands to the United States of America in 2000 was a shock, as I couldn't work until I received a work authorization card. With lots of time, I started to write a column for "Oedeminus", volunteered, and took more courses to increase my manual lymph drainage skills.

The happy ending is that I am working in America as a certified lymphedema therapist and I am still enthusiastic about it! Also, I have gone from writing a quarterly column to writing lymphedema articles, books, and stories such as this one.

I am glad that in this big country I can be of help. Not by keeping my finger in the dike to prevent flooding, but by using my experienced hands to drain lymphedema from the tissues!

Alma Vinjé-Harrewijn, PT, CLT

The Seams of Life

"When we consider the Circle of Life, every circle is unique and very special, no matter how the seams are sewn."

Editors' Note: In addition to being a busy therapist, Carol is a medical seamstress and develops creative solutions for patients. Join Carol as she creates custom solutions for compression problems.

As a Certified Lymphedema Therapist, I have been treating patients with lymphedema for more than eight years. Prior to treating lymphedema patients, I enjoyed being a therapist to burn patients for 13 years.

I am an Occupational Therapist who has developed a special interest in making medical garments and devices. This specialization arose from my passion about being creative and having an intense interest in medical conditions.

It has been remarkable to me how these two diverse interests have come together to allow me to be an artist and a caregiver in one!

In my practice, when I look at each medical condition or situation referred to me for evaluation, I see a unique opportunity. Sometimes I realize that the most logical solution is to explore the ready-made products that are available for purchase. This is an easy and usually less costly solution, and I employ this as often as possible.

If the ready-made solutions are not out there, I get my creative thinking cap out of the cupboard and go to work.

Usually my task is about coming up with a garment that provides compression on an extremity or body part in a way that enhances the ability of the lymphatic system to drain into functional lymph vessels. Being knowledgeable about the lymphatic system is imperative in the design and fabrication of garments.

Knowledge about fabrics and accessories are also important, as this allows flexibility in design and comfort. Understanding the impairment is paramount in designing and fabricating any garment or device. Therein lies the challenge. The wheels are turning in my brain. In my mind's eye I am seeing the types of materials I can use. I am assessing the person's ability to safely and comfortably be able to apply and remove the garment/device. I am learning about the lifestyle of the person for whom I am designing.

My goal is that they will be comfortable wearing the garment/device as prescribed, and I am always aware of the lifestyle changes that must take place for the patient to be successful in using the garment/device.

My supplies, fabrics, scissors, and a special serger sewing machine designed for sewing stretchy fabrics, are kept in our sewing room. I generally have a basic pattern in my head or in my file. Then I take very specific and accurate measurements so that the pattern can be drafted on my tracing pattern paper.

I love the feel of the paper and always start with a sharp pencil so my patterns are clear and precise. Then, as the pattern begins to emerge, my excitement grows!

As I lay out the fabric, it is just flat material on my cutting table. But when I put the pattern down, I begin to see the emergence of a "life" in its infancy. CUT, CUT, CUT go the scissors. The whirring sound of the sewing machine means that the garment is about to take a shape and become a real "life-improving" apparatus. SEW, SEW, SEW goes the machine, then the snipping of the threads as they hang at the beginning and end of seams.

I am aware of the many adjustments I must make in my posture to accommodate the growing "baby." I am using many fingers to hold the fabric as it serges under the pressure foot of the machine. Sometimes I catch myself with my tongue sticking out of my mouth onto my lip and I hold my breath when I am making a particularly difficult seam (all of which are essential when being creative, I think).

The sewing progresses until I have a real true "life" in my hands. It has taken the shape of the initial idea and my hope is always that it will be a perfect fit. But, like life, not everything is perfect, and adjustments have to be made so that the goal can be achieved. We want this "life" to be comfortable so that it fits into the lifestyle that we desire. So I place the garment/device on my patient, discuss the way it feels, look at the fit, analyze the compression, and make adjustments.

Sometimes I have to rip out seams, and go back to the sewing machine many times in order to "make it fit" (as my dear mother often said when teaching me to sew). But when it fits, and the "baby" has become a "life-improving" apparatus, then I sigh a breath of relief and know that it has become a second skin that performs its duty as it was designed, to keep lymphedema under control.

Having a goal and a vision is part of the process. However adjustments are always necessary in everything we do; we don't always get it perfect and it doesn't always turn out the way we envisioned it.

Adjusting and adapting to changes is a constant in our lives, and accepting this had made my role as a caregiver and artist very rewarding. When we consider the Circle of Life, every circle is unique and very special, no matter how the seams are sewn.

Carol L. Johnson, OTR/L, CLT-LANA

Chapter **3**

Learning about Lymphedema

Editors' Note: These contributions cover various aspects of how people get a lymphedema diagnosis and learn about lymphedema and its treatment.

We're delighted that you are reading about lymphedema and learning through sharing others' experiences. After all, it's your body and your life. You have a right to know, to understand, and to speak up for what you need.

The First Step

"It is up to the patient to be proactive about their condition and to demand further research into a solution."

Editors' Note: Lymphedema therapist Elizabeth Shapiro shares her thoughts on taking action to obtain diagnosis and treatment.

Everything we do in life, all of the endeavors we try to accomplish, begin with that first step towards a goal. All goals are attainable with drive and the proper support system.

When we feel sick, or have a feeling that something is wrong with our bodies, we turn to doctors and other medical professionals for help, support, and direction. Sometimes we are steered in the wrong direction, but it is up to the patient to be proactive about their condition and to demand further research into a solution.

I see patients every day who have struggled to get to the root of their swelling. They have been to countless doctors: cardiologists, internists, podiatrists, vascular doctors, orthopedic surgeons, and neurologists—just to name a few.

These patients are often put through extensive testing such as MRIs, CT Scans, venous Doppler ultrasound exams, and sonograms—all to no avail. All of this to try to get an answer to the question, *"Why am I swelling, and how can I get rid of it?"*

A common occurrence is for a physician to say, *"Elevate your legs and see me in a week."* Has this happened to you? If it hasn't, fabulous! If it has, there is help for you! If a part of your body feels swollen or congested, you may need to see a lymphedema therapist as soon as possible.

Lymphedema therapists are people who have dedicated their lives to educating others about lymphedema, preventive measures, and therapeutic interventions. It is up to you, as the patient, to push your physicians to become educated about lymphedema and treatment options available.

Before you can be treated by a lymphedema therapist, you must obtain a written referral from a physician. If your doctor is reluctant, it is up to you, as an educated patient and your own advocate, to push your doctor for this referral, at least for a consultation.

In my experience, a proper diagnosis is often harder to obtain than treatment for lymphedema. Once you have received a diagnosis of lymphedema, the prospect of decreasing your swelling and pain, and increasing your quality of life, is right around the corner.

When you see your doctor for a diagnosis, there are a few things that should happen.

A clear family history should be discussed. If your great grandmother always seemed to have swollen ankles, tell the doctor! If you are a poor historian, bring someone along who can help you.

A medical history will be taken. Even if it happened years ago, be sure to tell your doctor if you have had cancer treatment, surgery, an accident, or serious burn. Anything that can cause scaring or tissue damage might cause lymphedema.

You will want to discuss your symptoms with the doctor, and answer all questions to the best of your ability. It is a good idea to create a written medical history to take with you to the doctor's visit. It is much easier to remember all of those events and dates when sitting quietly at home.

The physician will be likely to inspect your swelling, making note of your skin integrity, look for signs of infection or for anything else that may lead them to believe you have lymphedema.

It is likely the doctor will palpate (touch/press) your skin to check for signs of edema. When the doctor pushes a finger against the swollen tissue and it leaves an indentation, this is known as pitting edema and is a diagnostic sign for the presence of lymphedema and the condition of the skin (or stage).

In some instances fluid retention is so severe that the skin appears to be bursting or weeping (leaking fluid), and the physician will automatically know.

You may hear the doctor say *"You have stage 3+ pitting edema,"* don't be alarmed. The stage 3+ is a standard gauging system for the severity of the edema and the condition of the skin. Nothing to be afraid of! Most edemas are resolvable with lymphedema therapy and patient compliance.

As a lymphedema therapist, I urge you to spread the word about what you know about lymphedema. Create networks among your peers and family to educate others about lymphedema. For those with lymphedema, diagnosis is the first step to a healthy life.

Elizabeth Shapiro, MS, OTR/L, CLT

Getting a Diagnosis and Finding Treatment

"If you suspect lymphedema, and your doctor is not sure, you can request a referral to a lymphedema therapist for a consultation."

Editors' Note: Sometimes finding treatment is a case of "Let the buyer beware". Mary Pat offers her suggestions and some cautions.

The more you know about what constitutes effective treatment and appropriate lymphedema therapist training, the more likely it is that you will get the effective help you deserve.

Getting Diagnosed

It is estimated that 90 percent of all lymphedema cases can be diagnosed on the basis of the patient's medical history and current symptoms. The remaining 10 percent of cases require more complex diagnostic testing.

Under law, only a physician can diagnose lymphedema (or any other medical condition). Unfortunately many doctors are unfamiliar with the condition.

When someone suspects they have undiagnosed lymphedema and is not getting anywhere with their doctors, I suggest finding a doctor who is knowledgeable about lymphedema and refers patients to qualified therapists. The question is: "How do you find that doctor?"

One thing I recommend is contacting a qualified lymphedema therapist and asking for the names of doctors they recommend, or doctors from whom they get accurate lymphedema referrals. Lymphedema therapists cannot legally diagnose you or treat you without a referral, but they sure know who is doing a good job of sending them patients with lymphedema.

If your doctor is uncertain about a diagnosis of lymphedema, you can request a referral to a lymphedema therapist for a consultation to help confirm, or rule out, possible lymphedema.

Finding Treatment

After lymphedema is diagnosed, the patient's doctor needs to write a prescription for treatment. A lymphedema therapist cannot begin treatment without this. A patient may need to be insistent about being referred to a qualified therapist.

Locating a therapist is often a matter of asking for recommendations and referrals. Potential sources of this information include cancer support groups, rehabilitation programs, oncology practices and breast cancer programs. Not all forms of lymphedema are associated with cancer. A qualified therapist is trained to treat both primary and secondary lymphedema.

Who Is A Qualified Lymphedema Therapist?

Ah, but who is a "qualified" therapist?

A qualified lymphedema therapist is trained to provide all phases of Complete Decongestive Therapy (CDT) including manual lymph drainage (MLD), the appropriate use of compression, and instruction in patient self-care techniques.

Those of us with lymphedema are dependent on our therapists for our wellbeing and quality of life. This is why it is useful to be aware of the training standards for a qualified lymphedema therapist.

Educate yourself by learning what is required to be a qualified lymphedema therapist. The basic standard for a Certified Lymphedema Therapist (CLT) as defined by the Lymphology Association of North America (see page 219) requires a medical license, specific college level courses, and 135 or more hours of postgraduate training in Complete Decongestive Therapy. CLT-LANA or certification by the Lymphology Association of North America is a more advanced qualification that also requires supervised experience, successful completion of a standardized exam, and continuing education to maintain certification.

After you know the recommendations for training, ask your therapist if he or she meets them. If not, it is time to search for a qualified therapist.

Some estheticians offer lymphatic massage to enhance the health and well-being of their clients. Estheticians are **not** licensed health care professionals and their training does not cover Combined Decongestive Therapy, lymphedema care, or other medical applications of manual lymph drainage. Lymphatic massage is no substitute for the treatment and care provided by a qualified lymphedema therapist.

When interviewing a new therapist never be shy about making inquiry about the therapist's qualifications.

Mary Pat B.

Chronic Venous Insufficiency and Lymphedema

"Treatment reduces the swelling and symptoms, helps to prevent complications of ulcers and infections, and improves the tissue texture of the legs."

Editors' Note: Anna Kellogg explains a common cause of lower extremity lymphedema that is not related to cancer treatment or injury.

Secondary lymphedema is most commonly associated with lymph node removal as part of cancer treatment. As therapists, we often see individuals with lymphedema in the legs caused by chronic venous insufficiency (CVI). CVI can occur when the veins are not effectively transporting blood up out of the legs because of weakened valves. The lymphatic system tries to compensate for this by absorbing and transporting extra fluid from the tissues. Eventually the lymphatic system becomes overwhelmed and is no long able to compensate for the insufficient venous system, at this stage the swelling of lymphedema develops.

Risk factors for CVI include heredity, obesity, pregnancy, smoking, being a woman and over 50, and jobs that involve prolonged sitting or standing. CVI can also be associated with deep vein thrombosis or blood clots, as well as venous ulcers. Besides the ankles and lower legs being swollen (edematous), individuals may have subjective symptoms which include the legs feeling achy or painful, tired or heavy. There may be visible varicose veins on the legs and the skin color may become darkened (hyperpigmented). The skin and tissues might change and have a shiny appearance or a thickened texture.

The treatment for lymphedema related to CVI is the same as for secondary lymphedema caused by cancer treatment. Treatment modalities include manual lymph drainage (MLD), compression bandaging and compression stockings, as well as skin care. The treatment reduces the swelling and symptoms, helps to prevent complications of ulcers and infections, and improves the tissue texture of the legs.

Anna Kellogg, OTR/L, CLT

Learn as Much as You Can

"Be an informed consumer."

Editors' Note: Here is some wonderful general advice from Tracy Novak of the West Virginia Lymphedema Network.

Learn as much as you can about lymphedema. Everyone with lymphedema should be an informed consumer and be prepared to be your own advocate.

We recommend studying **Living Well with Lymphedema** by A. Ehrlich, A. Vinjé-Harrewijn PT, CLT, and E. McMahon, PhD. This book, published by Lymph Notes in 2005, is available online through www.amazon.com.

Tracy Novak

Advice to the Lymph-Lorn

"Don't hide it from yourself; stoicism won't make it go away."

Editors' Note: Barbara lays it on the line in a bracingly no-nonsense style as she explains about lymphedema treatment. She has been living with primary lymphedema of the lower extremities (specifically Meige's disease) since 1961 but it was not until 2002 that the cause of her chronic swelling and inflammation was diagnosed and she began treatment.

Don't ignore symptoms of a problem.

None of us has a perfect body, but you know yourself well enough to know that swelling, pain, stiffness, heat and discoloration are not normal. Don't hide it from your spouse, partner, best friend, doctor, parents, or children. Above all, don't hide it from yourself; stoicism won't make it go away for you any more than it did for me.

Take care of your physical health.

If you don't smoke, don't start. If you do smoke, try to quit, or at least, don't smoke around me.

Keep your weight to a healthy minimum (no easy feat for many people!), eat (and drink) more foods and beverages that are good for you than that aren't, get as much low-impact aerobic exercise as you can (swimming and walking are the best; bicycling is wonderful, too), and wear clothing that's comfortable and appropriate for your needs.

If your lymphedema is in your lower extremities, as mine is, wear well-made, supportive shoes. Don't skimp on them.

Specialized lymphedema treatment—CDT, or complex (or comprehensive or complete) decongestive therapy—is essential. Period.

It's got to be the most obnoxious and archaic treatment in existence, and at least in my case, it doesn't provide complete or lasting relief. To a considerable extent, it only works while I do it. Maybe that's because I couldn't get the disease diagnosed for four decades. Whatever the case, I do it because I have to do it. So do you. Learn how to do it as independently as possible.

The treatment? I'll be honest here: I call it enslavement. Compression bandages and accessories; compression stockings, toecaps and special foam; exercises to pump the lymphatic fluid up from the toes and feet; constant protection of the feet and legs against scrapes, scratches, pinpricks, insect bites, injections, sunburns, heat, light. Good heavens, it never ends!

Does it get discouraging? Oh, yes. In fact, it gets infuriating, especially looking back on four decades without a diagnosis until finally learning that it is indeed a real disease.

And the fear of what it could do to me. That's all pretty scary. Sometimes, even after four and a half years in treatment, it seems unbearably scary.

Then I get home at night, and take off my shoes and stockings and toecaps and Komprex foam and look down at my legs, and cry for joy.

I have malleoli (ankle bones)! I have metatarsals (foot bones)! I have veins and tendons in my feet, ankles and lower legs, and mighty sexy legs, too. WOW!!!

And I have shoes that I can actually wear now because of the treatment. Lots of shoes. Good practical shoes, with good support, and plenty of good walking shoes—but SHOES. Normal shoes. Pretty shoes. At least two dozen pair, at last report.

Get information about the disease and those who are experts in its treatment.

Ask your librarians for information. Many clinics and hospitals now have patient-family information and education centers, use them.

The Mayo Clinic's site (www.mayoclinic.com) has one of the best-written descriptions of lymphedema that I've seen. Good websites include those of the National Library of Medicine (www.nlm.nih.gov) and a number of sites dedicated to lymphedema: Lymph Notes (www.lymphnotes.com), the

National Lymphedema Network (www.lymphnet.org), the Lymphatic Research Foundation (www.lymphaticresearch.org), and Lymphedema People (www.lymphedemapeople.com).

Subscribe to groups and listservs like the Yahoo! lymphedema groups; they're free and informative. Go to www.yahoo.com and click on Groups or Health for information.

Take care of yourself as a whole person.

Lymphedema and/or other chronic conditions might determine much of your day-to-day life, but it isn't everything about you. Never be ashamed of taking care of yourself.

Do you paint, draw or sculpt? Is your lymphedema in your arms? Learn ways to deal with it without giving up your art. I know a man with Meige's disease who loves to play volleyball. That's certainly high-impact, but he keeps his weight down, so should he give up something he adores?

My colleagues and I enjoy crossword puzzles; I love to write; I enjoy reading mystery novels. Enjoy time with your friends and families. Do you have a pet? Enjoy your time together. I have two cats; they have their claws; occasionally one of them will poke me, and I panic; but I keep first-aid equipment handy and I use it when Charlotte (my cat) gets too playful.

Do you love music? I do, and I've been singing in choirs and choruses for many years. It gives me hope and joy and the opportunity to give both to others.

Barbara Pilvin

Learning to Live with Lymphedema

"I have learned many ways to live better with my lymphedema."

Editors' Note: Caring for lymphedema can be a balancing act. Marcene shares what works for her when she has a sudden swelling.

I am a 22-year breast cancer survivor and have had diagnosed lymphedema for 10 years. I advocate good continual maintenance care for all lymphedema patients.

By keeping up with the new knowledge and information on lymphedema and doing all maintenance care lymphedema requires, my arm is now stable and I am doing great—that is until lymphedema decides to "act up" with an infection or sudden swelling. (See page 209 for signs of infection, page 130 for tips on treating infections, and page 123 for first aid in the kitchen.

The causes of "acting up" can be overuse, flying (without proper compression), heat, or from what appear to be unknown causes.

After an infection has cleared, it is back to more time in the bandages, more rest, MLD, etc. until the lymphedema can come down again.

I have learned many ways to live better with my lymphedema by reading and talking with others.

Marcene Johansson

Editors' Note: Marcene talks more about the benefits she's found through talking with others in Support Groups (page 152).

I Wish I Had Learned About Lymphedema Emergencies Sooner

"I think I am doing better now."

Editors' Note: Shari's experience demonstrates how important it can be contact your doctor quickly and to aggressively treat and monitor any cut or infection. See the guidelines for recognizing an infection in the Appendix (page 209), information on treating infections (page 130) and the article about First Aid in the kitchen (page 123).

You are the most important person on your health care team!

I wish I had found the Lymph Notes website weeks ago and read the emergency part much sooner. Six weeks ago I dropped a piece of firewood on my leg and skinned it. An hour later, it did the burning and itching thing and was leaking like crazy.

Within a week I had an ulcer and now, to make a long story short, I am now fighting an infected ulcer. It is painful, and ugly. Try wearing compression over one of those! Ooowwee!!!

I am now on my second bout of antibiotics. At one time I had a red streak going up my leg. I think I am doing better. Anyway, in the future I will get ahold of my doctor a lot sooner.

Shari Harper

Editors' Note: a red streak going up a limb indicates a life threatening infection. Seek emergency medical treatment immediately if you have any sign of an infection in an area that is affected by lymphedema, especially if you have had previous infections. Be sure and tell your regular doctor about all your infections.

If you do develop an infection, ask your therapist how to adapt your self-care routine and when you can safely resume self-massage and compression.

Frequently Asked Questions

Editors' Note: Because knowledge is power and there is so much misinforma-tion out there, we added this list of frequently asked questions about lymph-edema.

Q: "Will wrapping my leg in Ace bandages help?"

I have this swelling in my legs and it keeps getting worse. I've read about people wrapping with stretchy bandages to control swelling like this, but money is a problem for me. I'm considering buying Ace bandages from the drug store and wrapping my leg the way it shows in some of the photos.

Will this help?

A: Ace bandages are not a good idea!

Ace bandages, also known as long-stretch bandages, are used to relieve swelling and support a sprained joint. They are only used for lymphedema treatment in special situations (such as non-ambulatory patients) and can do more harm then good.

Specialized bandages, known as short-stretch bandages, are used in treating lymphedema. These bandages work on the principle of providing resistance to enhance the pumping motion of the muscles. It is this muscle pumping motion that increases the flow of lymph. Also, there are several layers of materials applied under the short-stretch bandages so that the wrapping is effective without damaging the circulation.

Starting to bandage for lymphedema is not a "learn-it-yourself" task. You really need to see a qualified lymphedema therapist for evaluation, treat-ment, and instruction. As part of the treatment your therapist will teach you the proper way to bandage (wrap) your affected limb based on your condi-tion. Once you've mastered this skill you should be able to self-bandage as necessary.

Q: Is it okay to wear a knit compression garment at night?

I have lymphedema affecting my legs. I'm doing well and am able to travel a lot on business. My problem is that my bulky night compression garments take up a lot of suitcase space. Would it be OK just to wear my knit compression hose at night?

A: No, it is not safe to wear compression garment at night!

Knit compression garments are made of specialized elastic knit with a two-way stretch that can be worn under clothing throughout the day, including while exercising. These compression garments are not to be worn while sleeping because they provide too much compression when the body is inactive. Also, if the garment moves out of place during sleep, it can cause constriction that damages the circulation.

See David Adcock's tips on compression at night, page 141.

Q: Can plastic surgery reshape my legs?

I've been to so many doctors looking for treatment of the lymphedema of my lower legs. It developed when I was a teenager and I'm now 39. I've been to many doctors without finding an answer; however, the last one suggested that I try the lymphedema clinic for treatment.

Instead of going through all that I was wondering, can't I just have plastic surgery to reshape my legs?

A: Plastic surgery will not solve the problem

Plastic surgery is not a cure for lymphedema. Plastic surgery may make your lymphedema worse by damaging the lymphatic vessels and creating scar tissue that makes draining the excess lymph even more difficult.

You will be better off if you follow your doctor's advice and seek treatment from a qualified lymphedema therapist. With treatment, it is usually possible to reduce the swelling and related problems, such as infections, and improve the condition and appearance of your legs.

Q: My doctor keeps giving me diuretics, are they helping?

My leg started swelling so I went to my doctor who prescribed a diuretic. The swelling keeps getting worse and every time I go back the doctor increases the dosage. Are diuretics helping?

A: Diuretics help for some things but not lymphedema

Diuretics can be effective treatment for edema of the legs that is caused by congestive heart failure, and for treating other conditions such as high blood pressure (hypertension). Diuretics are not effective for treating lymphedema in the absence of other conditions.

Swelling of the feet and ankles caused by congestive heart failure is not from damage or injury to the lymphatic system and is not lymphedema. Diuretics reduce this type of edema by stimulating the kidneys to remove more water from the bloodstream; this reduces the pressure in the venous system and allows the edema to drain from the tissues into the venous system.

Lymphedema is a disorder of the lymphatic system, not the venous system. Normally the lymphatic system transports protein molecules, cells, waste products, toxins, and even cancer cells out of the tissues, through the lymph nodes where they are filtered, and returned to the venous system. The swelling of lymphedema is excess lymphatic fluid that accumulates in tissues because the lymphatic system is unable to remove the fluid as quickly as it is produced.

Not only is removing water from the bloodstream not effective in reducing the swelling of lymphedema, it can make the condition worse and increase the risk of infection. When the fluid content of the body tissues is reduced by diuretics, two things happen. First, the protein in lymph attracts more fluid to the affected site and increases the swelling. Second, the proteins in stagnant lymphatic fluid become increasingly concentrated; this damages the tissues and increases the likelihood of a bacterial infection.

Check with your doctor to see why diuretics are being prescribed. See also the article on Chronic Venous Insufficiency and Lymphedema (page 72).

Q: How can I learn about taking part in clinical trials?

I've heard that there is research going on to see if drugs or complementary and alternative medicine can be effective in treating lymphedema. I'm anxious to do anything I can to help find better treatment or a cure for this condition. How can I take part in clinical trials?

A: Taking Part in Clinical Trials

If you are interested in learning about, or taking part in a clinical trial, go to ClinicalTrials.gov (www.clinicaltrials.gov) and search for "lymphedema." A list will come up of current clinical trials that are taking place around the world. The list includes information about the status of the clinical trial such as whether or not they are currently underway.

The Lymphedema Family Study is not a clinical trial but it is still an important opportunity for people with primary lymphedema to support research into the genetic factors in primary lymphedema, causes of the disease, and new strategies for treatment. Families in which two members have been diagnosed with primary lymphedema may be able to participate. For more information call the University of Pittsburgh at (412) 624-4657 or (800) 263-2152 or e-mail genetics@pitt.edu (be sure to include the words LYMPHEDEMA or GENETIC in the subject line of your message).

Chapter 4

Activities

Editors' Note: One theme running through so many of the stories is staying active and finding ways to continue activities that you enjoy, adapting as needed. You'll find lots of ideas in this chapter as well as in the next chapter on Travel.

Have you adapted your favorite activities so that you can continue them despite lymphedema? If you had to find alternative activities, what replacements have you discovered? Send us your story and we may include it in future versions of the book. We would love to hear from you.

Activities We Enjoy

"I try to maintain my lifestyle and pay attention to what my body is telling me."

Editors' Note: This list started as a survey of West Virginia Lymphedema Network members and now includes suggestions from other contributors and Lymph Notes members.

The activities listed here show the variety of interests and activities that are possible despite lymphedema. Although not all are suitable for everyone with lymphedema, the comment heard most often is: "I am not limited because I modify the activities to accommodate my lymphedema." How many of these activities have you tried and enjoyed? Caution: Please remember that this list of activities is not a "one size fits all" recommendation. Some activities may not be safe for you, depending on the extent of your lymphedema and other health factors.

Check with your lymphedema therapist and other health care providers if you feel inspired to try something new and strenuous, or if you have any questions about appropriate activities. We wish you happiness and good health.

- Aerobics

- Biking: bicycling at the gym or outdoors, motorcycle riding, mountain-biking, and riding a recumbent bicycle

- Bird watching

- Boating: rowing, kayaking, sailing, dragon boat racing, and "paddling anything that floats"

- Cardio machines

- Caring for animals: cats, chickens, dogs, goats, horses, and "almost anything with fur or feathers"

- Church and family activities

- Computer-related activities: playing computer games, searching the Internet, and selling stuff on e-Bay

- Cooking: gourmet, bar-b-que, and competitive

- Crossword puzzles

- Dancing: "All kinds, you name it and I'd love to try it!"

- Exercising

- Family time with children, grandchildren, and extended family

- Fun with my friends, including shopping!

- Gardening

- Golfing, see Jeanette's story on page 97.

- Handcrafts, photography, pottery making, scrap booking, sewing, and woodworking

- Hiking, see Jayah's story on page 12.

- Hockey

- Learning foreign languages

- Listening to music

- Outdoor Activities: backpacking, camping, deep sea diving, fishing, hiking, horseback riding, hunting, snorkeling, and surfing. See Tracy's backpacking story on page 93.

- Painting: watercolor, acrylics, and house

- Pilates, see Naomi Aaronson's story on page 91.

- Playing an instrument: bouzouki, guitar, and ukulele

- Pole-vaulting

- Reading

- Researching genealogy

- Running, including marathons, see Anna Kennedy's story on page 95.

- Singing: barbershop quartet, choir, karaoke, and solo

- Soccer

- Spirituality, see Brent's story on Self-Care and Mediation on page 136.

- Sudoku puzzles

- Swimming

- Tai Chi, see Emily P. Bees' story on page 91.

- Tennis

- Traveling abroad or domestically, exploring the country, RV'ing, and visiting historical sites. See the Travel chapter starting on page 103.

- Ultimate Frisbee

- Volunteering: on 4-H projects at our community center and at the senior center

- Walking: mall walking, Nordic walking, walking outside, walking on the treadmill

- Water aerobics or other aquatic exercises; see Mary Pat B. (page 99) and Mary Essert (page 100).

- Weight-lifting

- Working: as a lymphedema therapist, mail delivery person, school bus driver, teacher, or teacher's aide

- Writing

- Yoga, see Jennifer's story on page 89.

How Lymphedema Affected My Athletic Activities

" It was to my great relief that I was able to continue, and take pleasure in, my favorite forms of exercise."

Editors' Note: So many of our contributors were eager to share ideas on how to continue, alter, or replace activities. The message, over and over, is that you can be active despite lymphedema. Here's how Brent adapted his exercise routine.

One of my great apprehensions with the onset of lymphedema was that my ability to exercise would be seriously hampered. Throughout my adult life, exercise has been a vital part of my daily routine and a support for my physical and emotional wellbeing.

Some medical professionals told me that I should exercise less; others advised me to simply be attentive to the state of my body and the messages it was sending.

I opted to continue to exercise as I always had: biking for about an hour each day in my commute to work, swimming three times a week, lifting weights, using an exercise bike, stretching, and dancing.

It was to my great relief that I was able to continue, and take pleasure in, all of these forms of exercise. I have experienced some restrictions in my exercise, but these have not been major.

My kick in swimming is a bit slower due to reduced ankle flexibility. I have been in dance classes where I cannot perform some moves the same way that everyone else does. I need to take breaks in a workout to elevate and massage my leg for a few minutes.

When cycling at the gym I discovered that I prefer to use a recumbent bike instead of an upright one. On a recumbent bike, the rider lies back in the seat instead of being perched on top. I have found that this puts my legs in a higher position that is more beneficial for exercising legs affected by lymphedema.

I mentioned this to my vascular surgeon. His comments were that it makes sense to have the legs as high as possible and it helps reduce the swelling.

Recumbent bikes are found in some gyms and physical therapy facilities. They are also sold for bicycling outdoors on the road.

When I'm not at the gym, I have found that lying on my back and doing vigorous bicycle kicks in the air for a few minutes is one of the best exercises for loosening the lymph in my leg.

One of the largest hurdles for me, in coming to terms with the lymphedema was changing into and out of my compression legging in the locker room at the gym. When I started, this was challenging for my ego—as was having to change from using a brief swimsuit to something much larger and looser.

I maintain a strong sense of gratitude that I am able to engage in and enjoy all the athletic activity that I take part in.

I have been fortunate in having had, throughout my adult life, a strong sense of happiness in being embodied. This sense has allowed me, even with the lymphedema, to have an overall positive sense of my physicality and pleasure in my body.

Brent

Yoga—the Gentle Exercise

"Allow your body-mind to absorb the benefits of your practice and to tap into its own natural healing process."

Editors' Note: Jennifer explains why she recommends yoga and shares her tips on getting the most benefit from it.

According to Jane Verdurmen Peart, a yoga instructor at Stanford Cancer Supportive Care Program, "Yoga is beneficial in managing lymphedema because the deeper state of relaxation achieved through yoga has a positive impact on the lymphatic system and practicing yoga keeps the fluid pumping through the body.

"Also the yoga breathing practices promote lymph flow by strengthening the diaphragm and its movement, which creates an internal massage for the lymphatic vessels."

The following suggestions, which were gathered from several sources, contain helpful information for planning your practice of yoga:

- Work with a qualified yoga teacher who is knowledgeable about lymphedema. Possible sources of such teachers are centers that hold yoga classes specifically for cancer survivors. Also the Yoga Alliance web site provides helpful information and suggestions on how to find a qualified teacher. (www.yogaalliance.org)

- Always wear a compression garment or bandage during your yoga practice.

- Listen to your body and do not to over stimulate or tire the muscles. Muscle strain causes the muscles to tighten; this hinders lymph circulation and causes fluid buildup, which is exactly what you're trying to avoid.

- If you are getting tired or notice the beginning of an ache, rest, elevate the arm (or leg), and focus on the gentle expansion (inhale) and contraction (exhale) of the breath.

- Start with simple poses and gentle breathing which stimulate the lymph flow.

- If you are in a class that is not tailored to cancer survivors or people with lymphedema, it may be necessary for you to ask the teacher to modify the pose for you.

- If you are working on your own with a book or tape and a pose seems difficult, try going into the pose only halfway, or skipping it altogether, until you can get further instruction.

- Avoid the more strenuous types of yoga poses. The Headstand, Shoulder Stand, and Downward Dog place too much weight on the arms, neck, shoulders, and arms.

- Pay attention to conscious breathing during the poses. This increases their benefits.

- Rest and continue to pay attention to conscious breathing between poses. This helps your body to relax from the previous pose and prepare for the next pose.

- Take time for relaxing the breath for at least several minutes after your yoga practice. This is valuable for both body and mind. It also allows the body-mind to absorb the benefits of your practice and to tap into its own natural healing process.

Enjoy!

Jennifer

Consider Tai Chi

"The concentration and gentle stretching movements can relieve some lymphedema symptoms."

Editors' Note: Emily likes Tai Chi. Discover why.

I enjoy doing Tai Chi, but I've never felt certain that it helps with the lymphedema. On the other hand, it might help some people and the long slow movements are easy to do. I've seen people who had to sit in chairs doing Tai Chi. So, with the right instructor, it certainly is a form of exercise that is available to just about anyone.

There is little research on Tai Chi and lymphedema. I did find one article in *CancerWise* (the newsletter of the MD Anderson Cancer Center) reporting that the concentration and gentle stretching movements involved in practicing tai chi may help relieve some of the symptoms of lymphedema and another in *Supportive Care in Cancer* reporting that showed that Tai Chi Chuan had a positive effect on health-related quality of life for breast cancer survivors.

Emily P. Bees

Pilates Exercises

"Pilates is gentle to the body while giving it a challenging workout."

Editors' Note: Naomi discusses her reasons for recommending Pilates and shares general advice about exercising safely with lymphedema.

"*Recovercises for Wellness*" is a specialized program that I teach to help speed recovery from breast cancer surgery and to prevent the development of lymphedema. When I started working with breast cancer survivors in 1997, there was limited knowledge and research regarding lymphedema. At that time these women were told not to lift more than five pounds and they were scared. How could they get back to their daily lives and regain function and strength?

When one of my patients was diagnosed with lymphedema I didn't know what kind of exercise would help her. Since I knew so little, I attended classes to learn as much as possible and we have come a long way since that time!

Pilates is one of the exercises I've found that is a wonderful modality to incorporate in an exercise regime because it involves activation of the deep core muscles and deep breathing that stimulates the lymphatic system.

Pilates is unique because many of the exercises are performed lying down in a gravity reduced or eliminated position. Thus, one does not have to stand. Instead you can exercise in a supine (lying face up), prone (lying face down) or side lying position.

As when undertaking any new exercise program, there are important precautions to be observed when beginning Pilates:

- Always obtain doctors clearance before participating in any new exercise program including Pilates.

- If you have recently had a TRAM flap breast reconstruction, the abdominal Pilates exercises may not be appropriate for you right away. Get clearance from your surgeon before undertaking this program.

- Also before undertaking Pilates, it is important to obtain a baseline bone density test (DEXA) to determine if you have bone thinning (osteoporosis) or low bone density (osteopenia). Certain Pilates exercises require bending and twisting movements of the spine that are **not** recommended for anyone with either of these bone density conditions.

- Work with a Pilates practitioner who has experience with the special issues faced by breast cancer survivors, lymphedema patients, and individuals with bone density problems. Increasingly occupational therapists and physical therapists are learning Pilates and their professional background is oriented towards proper body mechanics and rehabilitation. A well trained and experienced Pilates practitioner should be able to adapt or change the exercises to meet your needs. Be aware that there is no regulation of Pilates and it is important that you ask a potential instructor about his or her background, training, and experience.

- Because the support it provides is essential, always wear a well fitted compression garment when exercising.

- Take individual lessons before joining a Pilates group. In the individual sessions you should learn the basics such as neutral spine, breathing and control before embarking on group sessions where you may not get as much supervision.

- Nothing should be painful. If an exercise hurts, speak up and ask the instructor to modify that the exercise to suit your body!

- Release unwanted tension from the body prior to starting each session. Pilates should be relaxing, yet you should feel energized, alert and stronger after participation.

Naomi Aaronson, MA OTR/L, CHT
www.recovercisesforwellness.com

Backpacking and Lymphedema

"When I developed lymphedema, I thought that I would not be able to backpack any more."

Editors' Note: Travel along with Tracy as she finds ways to resume backpacking. She doesn't let lymphedema keep her from doing what she loves.

Living successfully with lymphedema is a balancing act between being active without overdoing and making the condition worse. The following are the steps I took that made it possible for me to successfully go backpacking with the Boy Scouts!

When I developed lymphedema at the age of 41 as a result of breast cancer surgery, I thought that I would not be able to backpack any more because of this condition.

As I became more educated and more confident with my ability to manage my lymphedema, I decided last year to go on a short overnight trip with my 12-year-old son's Boy Scout troop. We hiked seven miles the first day. I think my pack weighed about 27 pounds. The second day was only a few miles hike back to the truck, but it was all straight up to get out so it felt a little longer than it was.

I did not have any increased swelling after the trip. (I know this because I keep a measurement diary and I measure several times a week.) I would like to offer some tips that I think helped me:

- As always, I wore my compression garment on my (affected) right arm.

- It was not a hot, humid, weekend when I took the backpacking trip. I think this made a big difference. It was rather cool and rainy.

- At no time did I really push it hard enough to overheat. I hiked at a pace that was very comfortable, even though we had quite a few big climbs. I also trained for a few weeks before going so I would not overheat as quickly and so I would feel strong for the hike.

- I used a hiking stick so that my hand/arm was always elevated while I was hiking—as opposed to just hanging down and swinging while I walked. I think this helped a lot.

- I did not lift my pack with my affected right arm. I always lifted the pack up with my left arm.

- I kept my right hand and arm elevated as much as possible. When we stopped to rest, I usually kept holding my hiking stick to keep my hand and arm elevated.

- I slept with my arm elevated. I put my backpack next to me in my tent and slept on my back with my arm elevated on the backpack.

- I carried several doses of penicillin with me as a precautionary measure in case I cut or burned my right arm. That way I could immediately start treating myself to prevent any kind of infection in my arm.

I did the same trip this year and again I did not have any swelling. I used all the same techniques except I wasn't able to elevate my arm at night because I was sharing a tent and there was no room for my pack. Again, it was not a hot, humid weekend; it was sunny and cool, with rain at night.

I think the cool weather, the compression garment, and the hiking stick were the three main keys to my success.

I encourage those with lymphedema to try to stay active and not let lymphedema limit you any more than it has to. I struggle with depression on a regular basis but professional lymphedema treatment, education, self-management, and common sense can go a long, long, way in controlling your lymphedema.

Tracy Novak

Walk a Day in My Shoes

"To me, MBT really stands for My Best Trainers."

Editors' Note: And if you're inspired to take up walking, exercising, running marathons or traveling around the world, you'll want to have a pair of good, comfortable shoes. Anna shares her experience and recommendations.

MBT stands for *"Masai Barefoot Technology,"* but I like to think it stands for *My Best Trainers*—a shoe that is not only comfortable for my power walking, but that aids in my lymphedema management by stimulating the lymphatics.

When I was first diagnosed with lymphedema, a friend of mine who knew how avid a power walker I was recommended a shoe she had seen advertised in a local specialty shoe store that promised, among other things, support for venous disorders. The brochure claims the shoe technology helps improve posture, increase circulation and strengthen muscles. It seemed logical to me that perhaps the shoe could help my lower leg lymphedema as well. I was eager to try anything that might help promote lymph flow in a compromised lymphatic system and at the same time aid my power walking.

I have since learned that the Vodder Clinic in Walchsee, Austria—a world renowned in-patient lymphedema clinic, whose founder created manual lymph drainage—recommends the MBT shoe to all their patients. Furthermore, all the doctors, nurses and therapists in the clinic wear them as well. The MLD therapists wear them during treatments, rocking back and forth on the shoe while they provide the MLD therapy for patients. At this rate, both patient and therapist are getting a good workout.

I want to thank Dr. Kettenhuber of the Vodder Clinic for kindly taking the time to answer my question on why the doctors in their clinic recommend the MBT shoes to their patients.

"… the structure of the MBT shoe forces the patient/client to use the muscles in their legs, especially the calves. So the venous flow in the direction of the heart is better. Because the lymphatics react on exercise as well, this has a benefit for lymphedema patients." Dr. Kettenhuber goes on to explain that *"the main aim for the shoe is on the muscles of the calf, but the rest of the leg and the lower back are stimulated too. Proper instruction is necessary, with shoes being worn for two hours at a time initially and then gradually working up to all day wear … in general they are very good for lymphedema patients."*

Although the shoes are pricier than most regular sports shoes, they have outlasted several pairs of other specialized shoes I used for power walking. I consider them my lucky shoes not only because they are comfortable and at the same time stimulate my lymphatics, but because I wore them when I completed my very first half marathon event. The specially trained salespeople ensure that you are walking on them correctly before you leave the store and MBT provides an educational CD with the purchase of the shoes. To find out where you can purchase them in your local area, check out their website at www.Mbt-info.com.

Anna Kennedy

When Can I Play Golf Again?

"It is not necessary to rule out the possibility of returning to the game."

Editors' Note: Golfers want to golf; it's just that simple.

If you have lymphedema and you want to resume playing golf (or you're considering taking it up), read Jeanette's reply to this question from a golfer with lymphedema who is eager to return to the game.

Among women golf enthusiasts who have been treated for breast cancer a common question is, *"How soon can I start playing golf again?"* The concept that they may not be able to play again because of the risk of lymphedema, or actually having lymphedema, comes as a shock that is nearly as unwelcome as the original cancer diagnosis.

There is no single answer to this question; however it is not necessary to rule out the possibility of returning to the game. Training should be completed with the approval of your physician and under the supervision of a lymphedema therapist.

Everyone who has been treated for breast cancer is at risk of developing lymphedema in the adjacent arm. This risk remains with you for life. Those with lymphedema affecting the legs are also at risk because of the walking and standing involved plus the hip-leg motion while swinging the club.

Although we usually think of lymphedema as affecting muscles because of the swelling, it is important to recognize that the joints are also affected. Due to the tissue changes associated with lymphedema, muscles and joints do not always respond to stress and repetitive motion in the same way as tissues that are not at risk for lymphedema.

The following are recommended cautions when considering returning to golf:

- Work with your physical therapist to restore the necessary strength and range of motion to your arms. Be comfortable in this range before pushing ahead.

- If you have lymphedema, or are at risk of developing lymphedema, always wear a compression sleeve while practicing or playing.

- Wear sunscreen and insect repellent. Sunburn can damage the delicate skin and an insect bite can lead to a serious infection requiring treatment with antibiotics.

- Drink plenty of water. Staying well hydrated is important in maintaining good health; it is even more important when you have, or are at risk of, lymphedema.

- Don't rush your return to the game. Practice a few holes or strokes and build-up very carefully. Determine how your arm responds and listen to your body. Repetitive motions are particularly stressful to the muscles of your affected arm. Negative responses, such as swelling or pain, do not always develop immediately.

- Be aware that walking places added strain on your arms and shoulders. If you have always walked around the golf course, consider using a golf cart until you are certain that your body is ready to handle the walking again.

- Do not lift or carry heavy loads with the affected arm. Handle your golf bag with your unaffected arm.

I'm not ready for tournament play (but then I never was); however, I am enjoying being back in the game again.

Jeanette, no longer a former golfer

Water Aerobics Are Fun

"I'm a water aerobics proselytizer. I admit it."

Editors' Note: Mary's message is that "Water, Water, Everywhere" is a good thing! Read on to find out why. Here is her story of becoming an enthusiast.

I'm a water aerobics proselytizer. I admit it. Being in the water is like being in full body compression. Serious movement while in the water makes it even better for me.

Partway through my initial lymphedema therapy, one of my knees started acting up. The physical therapist suggested water aerobics for the knee. It didn't sound swell to me, but the knee was really awful and I was ready to try almost anything. I figured I'd try it just to prove it wouldn't work.

Although it didn't heal my knee, it made it stronger and the recovery from surgery was much faster than it might have been thanks to the strength I'd gained. But it's not my knees that keep me in the water.

It's my lymphedema that keeps me in the pool—or maybe I should say it's my *lack* of lymphedema. After a few months of water aerobics, the lymphedema was very well controlled. It continues to be under control as long as I do water aerobics for an hour at least three times a week. I'm in the pool on my three "required" days and often on other days as well.

I found an instructor and group of classmates I really love. I prefer deep-water aerobics to shallow; keeping my shoulders in the water helps more. I've made some great water aerobics friends and the chance to see one another and to chat and laugh while we're in the water makes it easy to keep going.

For days when I can't go to class, I bought a waterproof MP3 player that I take into the pool to work out on my own. I play my favorite workout music or a cued water aerobics program with music and instructions. A good aerobic dance tape is fun and the moves can be adapted to the water. With lively music you have fun and feel better at the same time. I think the 70's era stuff works well for this.

Mary Pat B.

Aquatic Exercises for Lymphedema

"There are many benefits from being in water and exercising there."

Editors' Note: Here are thoughts, and cautions, from Mary Essert, a specialist in water exercises for those with lymphedema. Come on in, the water's fine!

For those with lymphedema, or at risk of developing it, there are many benefits from being in water and exercising there. These effects include:

- Being in the water is soothing, relaxing, and calming. It gives you a feeling of pleasure and wellness while reducing stress.

- The natural buoyancy of water reduces pressure on joints and relieves the negative effects of gravity on weight bearing muscles and bones. In chin-deep water you are 90% buoyant. This means that you feel only 10% of your body weight.

- Group aquatic classes provide pleasant social interaction. Everyone looks the same underwater so you may feel less self-conscious.

- The hydrostatic pressure of water against the body acts as a natural compression garment and aids in the reduction of swelling in the extremities. Hydrostatic pressure, which is the normal pressure of water against the body, increases the deeper you go into the water.

- Because of the ease of motion in the water, self-massage in water is more effective and is performed more easily.

- Deep abdominal breathing enhances the pumping in the thoracic duct and improves lymphatic drainage.

- Perform exercises in a pattern that follows the natural flow of lymph as it drains. Start with exercises that move the hands or feet and progress toward the trunk of the body.

- The comfort and ease of water exercise makes it easier for you to exercise regularly and to gradually increase the length or strenuousness of your water workout.

- The natural resistance of water makes exercise movements more effective. Because joints are supported, water also aids in increasing the range of motion.

- Exercising in the water strengthens muscles and improves muscle tone so that the muscles are able to stimulate the flow of lymph more effectively.

- Water exercises increase cardiovascular and respiratory fitness.

Precautions

- Consult with your healthcare professionals before starting any aquatic exercise program.

- A lymphedema aquatic exercise program should be performed in cooler water. Water temperature of 88° F is ideal. If the water is warmer, as in a therapy pool, the exercise should be for a shorter period of time using a shorter carefully individualized program.

- Start any new exercise program slowly and notice how your body reacts. One caution is that too much exercise may increase the amount of fluid to be pumped beyond what the heart is able to pump.

- Another concern is that muscle fatigue will not be obvious immediately and the effects of overdoing may not be obvious until later in the day.

- Do not go into the water, such as a public pool, if you have an open wound. It is particularly important that the skin be completely healed. Also apply lotion after the water session to protect the skin.

Mary Essert, BA, ATRIC

Mary is a water fitness specialist who develops and teaches therapeutic interventions for various conditions. For more information see www.maryessert.com.

Dragon Boat Racing

"This activity challenges the 'conventional wisdom' that a woman who has lymphedema must avoid strenuous activities."

Editors' Note: Hold on to your seats. Or perhaps we should say 'Hold on to your oars.' Here come the Dragon Boat Racers!

This is an inspiring example of women with lymphedema successfully challenging their limits.

The following information about the increasingly popular sport of Dragon Boat racing was provided by the Spirit Abreast Dragon Boat Team of Fraser Valley on their website (www.spiritabreast.com).

Dragon Boat Racing is colorful, hard work and a wonderful way to say, *"Yes I can!"* after breast cancer treatment. All over the world women who are survivors in every sense of the word are demonstrating their "can do" attitude as they take part in Dragon Boat Racing.

Dragon Boat racing has been part of the Chinese Culture for centuries and today teams around the world race colorful boats in heated competitions. During these races, each team member paddles hard to the beat of a drum. Despite any potential handicap, once in the race, the team competes on equal footing with other boats in their division.

This activity challenges the "conventional wisdom" that a woman who has had a mastectomy, or has lymphedema affecting the arm, must avoid strenuous activities. These teams have found that, **with appropriate precautions,** this can be very beneficial exercise. Also as the team trains and works together, they form an informal and closely bonded floating support group.

The teams, which consist of between 22 to 26 members, are made up of breast cancer survivors who range in age from 29 to 78. Special care is taken in their training to accommodate the needs of each team member. Teams train year-round both on land and in the boat and each paddler wears a support garment on the "at risk" arm.

Chapter 5

Travel

Editors' Note: Having just read about all the activities that people with lymph-edema engage in, it will not surprise you that it is possible to travel almost anywhere despite lymphedema, if you plan ahead.

Is It Safe to Go Around the World?

"Traveling with lymphedema is achievable and fun. It just takes a little more planning."

Editors' Note: Perhaps you, like Audrey, wonder whether it is safe to travel. She developed lymphedema after treatment for breast cancer three years ago. Now she wants to resume traveling, but she is uncertain.

Could she fly? For how long? What precautions should she take? What might happen if she pushed herself too hard? Here are answers provided by the Lymph Notes team.

Dixie's story of her trips to Brazil and Egypt and her travel tips follow.

For a long as I can remember, George and I have planned on traveling around the world after we retired. Unfortunately I was diagnosed with, and treated for, breast cancer three years ago and shortly after treatment I developed lymphedema. Now we wonder if it is safe for me to travel at all!

The dream lives on, but we need help in determining what is achievable.

Audrey

The Lymph Notes team did some research and found positive and practical advice for Audrey and George. Traveling with lymphedema is achievable and fun. It just takes a little more planning.

For each individual the starting point is to check with your physician and your lymphedema therapist. They should be able to provide clearance for take-off and valuable suggestions regarding your lymphedema and any other medical issues you may have.

Once you have been cleared to travel, here are essential precautions:

- Plan your trip for a leisurely pace that allows for rest periods if necessary. When you do too much you increase the chances of added swelling plus fatigue that takes the fun out of what you are doing.

- Include activities such as hiking and canoeing only if you are accustomed to this type of activity involving the affected areas. Remember that hiking affects the arms and shoulders as well as the legs. If in doubt, practice these planned activities at home before your trip.

- The National Lymphedema Network (NLN) position paper on Air Travel recommends that anyone with a confirmed diagnosis of lymphedema should wear some form of compression therapy (a compression garment or compression bandages) while flying; adjust the amount of compression to your needs, the length of the flight, and the altitude where you are staying. Individuals at risk for developing lymphedema should understand the issues associated with air travel and make an informed decision about compression based on their own medical history and condition.

- Avoid sitting in one position for long periods of time while flying or during other travel. Move your arms and legs frequently to prevent swelling; stand up and move around every 30-60 minutes, if possible.

- Stay hydrated by drinking plenty of safe water. This is particularly important in warm climates, arid areas, and during airplane flights.

- Follow your self-care routine as closely as possible every day while you are traveling. This includes self-massage, wearing a compression sleeve during the day and bandaging or wearing a compression garment at night. (Bandages take less space in your suitcase.)

- Take good care of your skin with sunscreen, lotion, and insect repellent. Something as minor as a bug bite can cause an infection.

- Remember your first aid kit. Treat any minor injury as if it were serious.

- Have your doctor write an antibiotic prescription and have it filled. Take these pills with you, in the original container with the pharmacy label in place. Should you develop an infection, take the medication according to your doctor's instructions.

- If you think you have an infection, don't wait. Cellulitis can spread and become serious very quickly! If you are going to make a mistake, make it on the side of taking the pills too soon.

- If you are a Medicare client, be aware that Medicare does not cover any medical treatment provided outside of the US. To get insurance coverage for emergency medical expenses outside of the US, be certain that your Medicare Supplement (Medigap) policy includes this coverage. All Medigap plans are required by law to have a $250 deductible on this benefit.

- If you are concerned about not being able to complete your trip, consider purchasing travel insurance that covers emergency medical care and trip interruption. Hopefully you won't need it!

Now the most important step! Relax, have fun and enjoy your journey.

My Trips to Brazil and Egypt

"I am not about to let lymphedema stop me from traveling and seeing the places I've always wanted to visit."

Editors' Note: As promised, here is the story of Dixie's trips to Brazil and Egypt. She shares her adventures (and misadventures) and the lessons she's learned. Where next? Kenya and Tanzania, there's no stopping her.

After gynecological cancer treatment, I now have secondary lymphedema affecting both legs. Controlling the swelling requires the diligent use of compression; however, I am not about to let this stop me from traveling and seeing the places I've always wanted to visit.

On one of my trips I traveled to a resort in the middle of the Pantanal in Brazil. The Pantanal is the world's largest freshwater wetland and one of the world's most productive habitats. It was said to be home to giant river otters, jaguars, marsh deer, and tapirs and I planned to see them all. I was also anticipating some spectacular bird watching since this wetland provides a natural habitat for more than 650 species of birds.

From the time I left home until I arrived at the resort, I traveled non-stop for 24 hours. This involved two long flights from the states, arrival at a tiny airport, and an additional five-hour jeep ride.

Usually when I travel on long flights, I wear padded leg garments with compression sleeves over them. The padded garments are necessary because wearing just knit compression garments on long flights doesn't work for me! Since this was an extremely lengthy trip I wanted even more compression and obtained this by adding a layer of bandages over the padded garments.

By the time I arrived, the bandages had been bunching at the knees for hours and were soaked with sweat due to the tropical heat. The result was a large collection of huge welts on the back of each knee. Frankly, I was scared! Here I was in the middle of nowhere and I was certain my legs were going to fall off. Medical care was hours away and I didn't know if it would be any good even if I could get to it. The best I could do was slather the welts with Neosporin and my jock itch medicine—and pray. Then, of course, I had to put on compression garments on again over that mess.

But it all worked! By the next day survival was assured and within two days—while still wearing my compression garments—all signs of that horror were gone. Whew! Now I was able to fully enjoy my surroundings.

Unless you live in the south, you may not be familiar with the minute and very nasty biting bug known as a chigger. Even when your legs are healthy, chigger bites can make life miserable with severe itching that is particularly bad at night.

I enjoyed exploring my surroundings and never gave any thought to the possibility of these critters. After all, I was well wrapped with breathable compression garments and I thought I was protected. These breathable garments were the logical choice for this trip because they are more comfortable in the heat.

What I didn't know was that "breathability" also means "permeability." I soon discovered this when my legs were bitten by chiggers. It is bad enough to have to wear these darn garments, the least they could have done was to provide protection from critters. Life is just not fair! However, I learned another valuable travel lesson: always take antihistamine cream or spray with you.

I had a fabulous vacation in Brazil, despite the chiggers, and too soon it was time to leave. I swapped addresses with my fellow bird watchers and we've extended the pleasure of our trip by swapping DVDs of our fabulous bird photos.

My next vacation trip was to Egypt. There were no chiggers there and—despite very hot temperatures—sweating problems were reduced because the humidity was low. Among my adventures on this trip, I even did the classic tourist activity and rode on a camel! With or without lymphedema, a camel would never be my favorite mode of travel.

This summer I'm off to explore Kenya and Tanzania and I can hardly wait! I'm certain there will be more adventures and many things to see. One thing is certain: No matter what happens, I do not intend letting lymphedema slow my travels!

Dixie Spiegel

Dixie's Travel Tips

"I have traveled for three weeks with very strict weight restrictions on my luggage and made out just fine."

Editors' Note: An enthusiastic world traveler, despite lymphedema in both legs, Dixie has a wealth of experience to share. She has not allowed lymphedema to slow her traveling, or lessen her enthusiasm! Here are her general travel tips.

Traveling with lymphedema does have some drawbacks, but it can be done. Just because this travel requires more planning, don't let lymphedema keep you from enjoying those trips you long for.

Here are some guidelines to help make traveling with lymphedema easier and achievable:

Wear Compression. The medical advisory committee of the NLN recommends that individuals with lymphedema wear some form of compression therapy (compression garment or compression bandaging) while traveling by air and that individuals at risk for lymphedema should decide based on their individual risk factors. For more information see the Air Travel Position Paper on www.LymphNet.org.

As an experienced traveler, I urge you to get compression garments that fit properly. A knit garment off the drug store shelf may only provide you with a false sense of security rather than effective compression. Your best bet is to consult a lymphedema therapist in order to obtain a properly fitted garment.

Save Suitcase Space. Padded compression garments and bandages for night wear could take up nearly an entire suitcase. Wearing these garments on long flights provides better compression and saves suitcase space, which you'll need for other lymphedema extras.

For very long flights, such as overseas, I wear my padded garments plus a knit compression garment to provide added compression. An alternative is to place a layer of bandaging over the padded garment.

Remember, What Goes Up, Goes Down. To save suitcase space, I travel in my padded Jovis (JoViPak garments). Since these don't offer as good long-term compression as my Class Four Plus stockings, I find it necessary to add extra compression by wrapping. Despite these precautions, sometimes when I arrive after a long flight my legs are swollen and resemble big, heavy tree trunks.

Working on the adage that, "What goes up (swells), comes down (is less swollen)", I get busy as soon as possible after landing. I remove the padded garments and replace them with my compression stockings. Then I lie down on the bed, and prop my legs up on the stacked suitcases. (At this point a nap feels good too.) Every night I do a good massage. Sometimes, particularly if I have been doing a lot of walking, I sleep with my legs propped up. Of course, it's annoying but it beats staying at home!

Make Thorough Lists. Unlike toothpaste, you can't generally find a replacement garment in Outer Mongolia! Start your list well ahead of your trip and keep it next to you as you go through your day with lymphedema. Revise your list as needed and then relax. If you follow your list, you will have everything you need.

Since I have to accommodate secondary lymphedema in both legs, your list may not be as extensive as mine; however, I know that I have everything with me. This is important because the stress of touring might increase my compression needs. Although the list is long, all of this really doesn't take up much space.

This is what my list includes:

- Three pairs of compression garments (my current pair and my two next least worn-out older pair) plus knee highs (because I may need that extra compression), extra toe pieces, and adhesive to help keep everything up. Don't forget the donning aids needed to get your stockings on and off.

- A bag to hold my padded Jovis when I am not wearing them. Straps are handy to compress the Jovis so they will fit in the bag. (Jovi is shorthand for a JoViPak brand padded compression garment that is usually worn at night.)

- Stockinette to wear under my Jovis at bedtime. I take six rolls of bandages just in case I need to give my Jovis an extra compression boost at night. I also take Artiflex or other padding in case I develop a hot spot that might develop into a blister. (Artiflex is a brand of felt-like padding that is routinely worn under lymphedema bandages.)

- Soap powder to wash my compression garments as needed. I also take two skirt hangers to hang up the stockings to dry. I've discovered that a few sheets of Febreeze fabric softener help to conceal the odor of Jovis that can get "really ripe" after three weeks in the tropics!

- Castor oil or other oil for massage plus a high quality hand cream to keep my feet smooth.

- Medications, including an antibiotic prescription in its original container, in case I develop an infection. Also include jock itch medications, antihistamine cream or spray to ease the itching of bug bites, sunscreen, and insect repellent.

That's a lot. Sure it is. But I have traveled for three weeks with very strict weight restrictions on my luggage and made out just fine. Let's face it: Most of us take way too many clothes on trips. Just leave out those two unneeded dresses and those three extra pair of shoes and you're good to go! And don't bring home so many tacky souvenirs that will just gather dust later.

<u>Plan Your Carry-On Carefully</u>. Luggage gets lost and delayed. With lymph-edema, you can't "make do" without your lymphedema supplies, even for a night. So make sure you have the minimum you need with you in the cabin of the plane. You don't have to smell good or be pretty, but you do have to be compressed!

<u>Don't Be Annoyed If You Get Singled Out By Airport Security</u>. In fact, I get annoyed when I am <u>not</u> singled out. Just imagine what I could have stashed under those padded Jovis! So far the most I have had to do is to let them lightly rub a special cloth over my Jovis to test for explosives. That took two minutes.

Dixie Spiegel

What to Wear While Flying—A Minority Opinion

"When we fly, I bandage my wife, Pearl, with short-stretch bandages."

Editors' Note: Exercising and drinking enough water while flying are clearly important. There are differing views on the use of compression and very little objective evidence. Bob Weiss makes a number of good points as he explains why his wife travels in short-stretch bandages. Dixie Spiegel's routine for flying involves more compression (page 108). The National Lymphedema Network's recommendation on air travel differ (page 104). Clearly more research is needed.

It is my (learned?) opinion that one should not wear an elastic compression sleeve when flying, any more than one would wear one while sleeping. Unless you can be doing continual or frequent exercise, the resting pressure of a compression sleeve is high because of the elasticity, and this would tend to reduce lymphatic flow instead of increase it.

Elastic compression garments such as the Medi, Juzo, Jobst circular weave, etc are made with elastic fibers that provide a high resting pressure and a low dynamic pressure. These are designed for use during the day, when the body is active and the leg or arm muscles alternately flex and relax. In so doing they aid in moving lymph. But when you are sedentary, this pumping is not effective. When you are resting at night or seated on an airplane they squeeze the arm continuously to increase the fluid pressure, and aid the flow of fluid into the venous system. In contrast, they may squeeze the lymphatic structures near the surface of the skin and block the flow of lymph.

Flat-knit garments such as custom Elvarex, Juzo Strong, Medi custom, etc. are better than the more elastic circular-knit garments. They exert less "resting pressure" and allow better lymphatic flow; however in both cases, you must exercise your arm. It is helpful to carry a sponge ball that you can squeeze during the flight, and to raise your arm above your head to let gravity help drain.

It is important in every case to exercise while in flight; however it is even more critical for lower-limb lymphedema because the limb is "dependent." With the lower limb, gravity pulls down on fluids (mostly venous fluids) and causes them to pool in the tissues. Exercise causes the circulatory system to provide better movement of blood, and this aids with lymphatic drainage too. I have the same comments about lower limb garments in flying as I do for upper limb. Best-to-worst is: bandaging or non-stretch garment, flat-knit, circular knit, nothing.

Also it is vitally important to travel with a well fitting graduated compression garments without any constrictions.

The frequent advice to wear compression during flying is a holdover from the days when swelling was believed to be a result of venous insufficiency blood pooling with the risk of thrombosis, and the graduated compression elastic stockings would raise distal to proximal tissue pressure, and enhance venous blood return to the heart. But the "squeezing" of a swollen limb to get rid of the fluid by venous return is not beneficial for pure lymphedema since it does little to improve lymphatic flow of the protein rich lymphatic fluid. These proteins then concentrate and due to their ability to attract more fluid they increase the swelling of the limb.

When we fly, I bandage my wife Pearl, with short-stretch bandages. These have a low resting pressure and high working pressure which enhances lymphatic flow when she does exercises on the plane. She brings a sponge ball which she squeezes rhythmically during the flight. She also does other exercises designed to use the muscle pump against the low-stretch bandages to move fluid out of her arm. Any request to unwrap the bandages is met with a request for a qualified lymphedema doctor to rewrap her. A detailed "wanding and sniffing" usually suffices. However we always travel with a set of rolled bandages and an Elvarex sleeve, just in case.

An alternate to bandages would be a non-elastic manually-adjustable sleeve such as the Reid Sleeve (very bulky for flying in), CircAid, or ArmAssist, which is our favorite for flying.

So my experience is at odds with the conventional recommendations, and there is no randomized clinical trial that I know of on this subject. But I believe that it is consistent with most analytical articles on the pathophys-iology of lymphedema.

Robert Weiss, MS
Lymphedema Treatment Advocate

Chapter **6**

Solutions to Common Problems

Editors' Note: When you have lymphedema you may have to be persistent and inventive. This chapter may give you some ideas to try and some great stories about finding answers to tricky problems.

For more ideas from our contributors on Self-Care Tips see Chapter 7.

When Treatment Is Too Far

"I live in a rural area, have a limited budget, and am unable to travel to a 'big city' for treatment. How can I get help?"

Editors' Note: Problems in finding, affording, and/or traveling to lymphedema treatment are common. Tracy Novak shares her pragmatic suggestions.

Here in West Virginia we often encounter the lament, *"I live in a rural area, have a limited budget and am unable to travel to a 'big city' for treatment. How can I get help?"* The following are guidelines we share with our West Virginia Lymphedema Network members who face this problem.

- **Realize that you need at least one session** with a qualified lymphedema therapist to help you get started with the self-care phase of lymphedema treatment.

- **You will need a prescription** from you physician before you make an appointment for this treatment. This usually reads, "For lymphedema treatment as needed."

- **Talk with the therapist by phone,** or e-mail before scheduling your initial treatment and explain your situation. Ask the therapist to set up a modified initial visit during which you will be taught the essential self-care skills (self-massage, bandaging, skin care, and exercises) that will enable you to provide basic treatment for yourself at home.

- **Arrange to have a family member or friend go with you** and attend the first treatment session as your "helper." The role of this helper is to learn the self-care skills and to make a video of the teaching portions of the treatment session or take detailed notes. If you don't have a video camera, you'll need to make arrangements to borrow or rent a video camera. Before your visit, ask the therapist for permission to have your helper video the training portion of your session.

- **If you have health insurance** or Medicare, determine what treatment will, and will not, be covered before you schedule appointments. Some policies will only cover one treatment per day. Some policies will pay for part of the cost of compression garments and bandages. Other policies do not cover this equipment and supplies. Insurance will probably not cover travel expenses for you or your helper.

- **At home,** and equipped with the necessary bandaging supplies, you and your helper should review your video and the information supplied by the therapist. Practice repeatedly until you are comfortable in this self-care skill.

- **Despite costs and distances,** it is a prudent idea to see your therapist at least once or twice a year. At this time progress is evaluated and it may be necessary to replace compression garments.

Tracy Novak

Surgery and Lymphedema

"Patients have to educate their doctors and the hospital staff."

Editors' Note: These stories by Mary Pat and Georgia (next) highlight the need for education, reminders, and precautions for protecting your at-risk limb.

Surgery brought on my lymphedema, so facing more surgery isn't a pleasant prospect. The first time around I was assured over and over that they would be very careful not to take blood pressure or use any needles on my "at risk" arm. Their intentions may have been good but I learned that many hospitals just don't have a protocol for being careful about this. I've since learned that some patients have signs over their beds about their lymphedema, but when you're being moved around the hospital there may be no protection.

I went into my first post-lymphedema surgery with my handy-dandy hot pink lymphedema hospital band (see the Editors' Note at the end of this story) on my wrist; however no one stopped to read it! Since hot pink wristbands were meaningless in that hospital, it got no respect at all.

I had to warn off several people pre-surgery regarding blood pressure cuffs, IV's, etc. During surgery the arm was wrapped and well protected, but as soon as I hit the recovery room someone was trying to put a blood pressure cuff on my "at-risk" arm. I was awake and able to ward her off, but most post-surgical patients are not that alert.

For my second surgery, I took the same precautions plus I had a neighbor write in large dry-marker on my arm "*Lymphedema, No Needles, No Blood Pressure.*" The surgeon, who knew about my concerns, was amused. I learned that sleeves on hospital gowns can cover everything from the shoulder to the elbow making it hard to read anything above the elbow.

I had better luck that time, but mostly because I kept talking about my lymphedema to everyone. Again, I was awake (spinal, no sedation) so I was able to defend myself when most surgical patients could not.

I'm now facing yet another surgery. I've told this surgeon about my experiences and the fact I feel they (doctors and hospitals) lack appropriate protocols for protecting surgical patients with lymphedema. The surgeon's suggestion was that I write on my arm again.

This time I'll write it twice—once above the elbow and once below. I'll tell everyone in sight about it (at least maybe I'll educate someone). And I'll have that well-used bright pink wristband for them to ignore.

I should be awake again to defend myself—but what a hassle. It irritates me that we have to go through this in order to have medical personnel to help us follow medical orders.

I think the only way things are going to change is for lymphedema patients to keep insisting over and over. Patients have to educate their doctors and the hospital staff. If these people hear it often enough, maybe they'll get the idea that they have a responsibility to lymphedema patients.

Mary Pat B.

Editors' Note: Hospitals use color-coded wristbands as visual cues to remind staff about critical patient information. Each hospital assigns its own colors and the meaning of a wristband color may vary between hospitals. Groups like the Color of Safety Taskforce are working on standards. Until we have effective standards:

- Your first choice is wristband provided by your hospital that indicates lymphedema or 'restricted extremity for blood draw.'

- If your hospital does not have an appropriate wristband, be sure that your lymphedema band does not conflict with, or hide, any hospital issued wristband.

- Remove any colored charity or social-cause bracelets that might cause confusion.

Peninsula Medical Supply offers free Lymphedema Alertbands for the wrist or ankle, see www.lymphedema.com.

The Sign on the Wall

"Lymphedema? I live with it, simple as that!"

Editors' Note: As Georgia's story demonstrates, sometimes even a sign over the bed or on the wall doesn't work!

I have had Lymphedema for seven years. I live with it, simple as that!

Here's what I remember. I woke up from having my mastectomy for the removal of my right breast. There in the recovery room, on the wall next to me, was a big old sign *"No Blood pressure taken on the right arm."*

Now, that sign was big—but where do you think my blood pressure cuff was? That's right, snug around my right arm.

Not being aware of the dangers of lymphedema, I asked the nurse, what that sign was for? Her eyes got big. She explained, and moved the cuff to the other arm.

That story has always stayed with me. It has taught me to be proactive about my arm.

Please do the same for yours!

Georgia Spidle

Pregnancy and Primary Lymphedema

"Primary lymphedema should not prevent you from having a family."

Editors' Note: Doris Laing shares her advice for women with lymphedema who are planning a family.

Since primary lymphedema (PLE) develops most commonly in women, it is only natural that questions about pregnancy arise. Many women, very wisely, are concerned about what to expect during pregnancy and how to manage it. I have worked with many PLE patients during pregnancy and have researched so I can effectively help my patients and be prepared to answer their questions and suggest precautions.

Here are precautions that can help you achieve these goals:

You Can Do It! Unless you have other health issues that make pregnancy risky having primary lymphedema should not prevent you from having a family. However, it is essential that your healthcare team work in close cooperation to help you achieve the goal of producing a healthy baby while protecting your affected leg(s).

Inform your obstetrician or midwife at your first visit. They need to know that you have primary lymphedema, or are at risk of developing it. Be prepared to supply them with information about lymphedema; suggesting a phone consultation with your lymphedema therapist can also be helpful.

Inform your therapist that you are pregnant. He or she should be an important part of your prenatal team by providing appropriate treatment, necessary advice, and recommended changes in your treatment and self-care routines.

Be extra cautious. A cellulitis infection is a danger to you at any time. During pregnancy, an untreated infection is a threat to you and your baby. Discuss this potential with your doctor and be prepared with emergency antibiotics.

Be an informed patient. Learn about how your body changes and ways in which the stresses of pregnancy can affect lymphedema. Also learn the danger signs that indicate you need to see your doctor as soon as possible.

Be prepared. As your pregnancy progresses you are going to need help with your self-care and possibly other routine activities. The time to recruit, and train, a helper or helpers is early in your pregnancy before this need is critical.

Manual Lymph Drainage is recommended throughout the pregnancy. This helps control the swelling and keeps you more comfortable. Additional treatments may also be necessary as the pregnancy places more stress on your body.

Continue your self-massage program. Maintaining self-massage on a regular basis is very important. As your pregnancy progresses and it becomes increasingly difficult for you to reach your legs and feet, this is the time for your "helper" to begin aiding with this routine. Also, ask your therapist for guidance in modifications of your abdominal breathing and massage for abdominal clearance as your pregnancy progresses.

Compression is a must throughout pregnancy. This routine can also need some modification to accommodate your increasing size. The exception to this is if, for any reason, your doctor instructs otherwise.

If you have been wearing compression panty hose before your pregnancy continue to wear them, unless you are told otherwise. Before investing in maternity compression hose, check with your therapist as to what level of compression is recommended.

If you were wearing thigh high compression hose be certain they do not bind. If this is a problem, ask your therapist for recommendations. Toward the end of your pregnancy, you may need help in getting these stockings on and off; here is another opportunity for your helper.

Bandaging: Even if you do not normally bandage, you may find it beneficial during pregnancy. This is because bandages have the advantage of being adjustable to accommodate changes in your leg size and the amount of compression that is needed. Bandaging your legs as your belly size increases can be challenging, if not impossible, to do by yourself. Again this is an opportunity for your helper

Skin Care: Pregnancy usually causes abdominal stretch marks and your OB or midwife may offer suggestions to minimize this scarring. It is also important to continue your proper lymphedema skin care—plus taking care of your feet and toenails. Again, you are going to need some help.

Walking Exercise: Exercise is very important for your general health, to promote a healthy pregnancy, and to control the swelling of your lymphedema. Walking is usually the preferred exercise and be sure to drink lots of water while doing this so that you do not become dehydrated. Seek your doctor's guidance in starting a walking routine and modify it as your pregnancy progresses.

Water exercises are excellent throughout your pregnancy. Toward the end of the pregnancy, as walking becomes harder, exercising and walking in the water become even more beneficial. Check with your doctor before heading for the pool, some doctors are concerned about how the chemicals in public pools might affect your body during pregnancy.

Bed Rest: You may find that in order to control the swelling you need to spend time on bed rest with your feet and legs elevated. This allows nature and gravity to help reduce the swelling. This is another area of your life where planning ahead and lining up some help can make this easier to manage.

Weight Control: Follow the recommendations of your healthcare team as to how much weight is healthy for you to gain. If you have a sudden weight gain (without binge eating) report this immediately to you doctor or midwife because this can be a sign of preeclampsia.

Preeclampsia is a rapidly progressive serious complication of pregnancy that affects both mother and child. It usually occurs after the 20th week (late second trimester) or in the third trimester. This condition is characterized by high blood pressure and the presence of protein in the urine. Swelling, sudden weight gain, headaches and vision changes are other important symptoms; however, some women with rapidly advancing disease report few symptoms.

The hypertension (high blood pressure) of preeclampsia puts an added strain on the heart and other body systems. To minimize strain on the heart, it may be necessary to modify the compression used to treat your lymphedema. Because of the added risk associated with primary lymphedema, your doctor may recommend monitoring of your blood pressure at home between visits.

If you develop any symptoms of preeclampsia, consult your doctor immediately. Your lymphedema therapist should also be notified because it may be necessary to modifying your bandaging and compression routines so they do not place excess strain on your heart and other body systems.

By following these precautions you increase your chances for a healthy pregnancy with a happy outcome. Best wishes.

Doris Laing, LMT, CLT-LANA

First Aid in the Kitchen

"Never apply hydrogen peroxide or iodine solution to an open wound."

Editors' Note: Even if we aren't professional chefs, most of us cook. Here are some useful tips in case of cuts or burns.

I'm a professional chef and I was treated a few years ago for melanoma of the arm. Not long after the surgery, I developed lymphedema in that arm. I've had a couple of infections and the most recent landed me in hospital.

During this miserable forced 'vacation' I realized that either I had to protect my hand and arm or find a new career! Once I got over my initial anger and fear, I came up with a plan with three parts. My recipe (this one is not a secret) calls for equal parts self-care, risk reduction, and effective treatment.

Self-care requires that I be more rigorous in self-massage, wrapping, and getting MLD treatments to keep the swelling down. As my therapist says, "Less swelling, less risk of infection."

Risk reduction is the hardest. I am traditional and stubborn so I'm used to doing things the old-fashioned way and very quickly. Safety has not always been a priority in our kitchen. We are becoming more safety conscious, slowing down a little, changing some of our methods, and paying more attention to accidents.

Treatment is another big change, most of what I had always done for first aid made my doctor cringe. We have a new first aid kit and new procedures; I now know to check daily for signs of infection and to seek medical treatment immediately for an infection or a serious injury.

Bleeding helps to clean out wounds, and most small cuts will stop bleeding in a short time. If the bleeding does not stop in a timely manner or the cut is large, seek medical care. After the bleeding stops, carefully clean the wound with mild antibacterial soap and water. An important rule that I learned is to never apply hydrogen peroxide or iodine solution to an open wound, these substances are toxic to the cells of a wound that is healing. Use a sterile Q-tip to apply an over-the-counter topical antibiotic cream, such as Neosporin over the wound and then cover it with a sterile bandage such as a Band-Aid.

If you bruise yourself on or near a lymphedema-affected limb, and the skin is broken, treat this injury as a cut or scratch. If the skin is not broken, reduce swelling and minimize discoloration by placing a cold pack, wrapped in a clean towel, on the injury. Keep this in place for no longer than 20 minutes at a time. Do not place ice directly over the injured area or apply ice to skin that is affected by lymphedema.

Burns are a major hazard in a busy kitchen and I quickly learned that the primary rule of treating burns is, "*Do not place butter, oil, ice, or ice water on burns.*" Beyond that, burns are treated according to their degree of severity and the amount of body area that has been burned.

For a first-degree burn that has no blisters or breaks in the skin, cool the burned area. Do this by applying a cold, wet, cloth for 20 minutes and then removing it for 20 minutes. Repeat this until the area is pain-free. Apply a low pH moisturizer, or an antibiotic cream, over the burn to prevent the burned tissues from drying out. Protect the affected area by covering it lightly with a dry gauze bandage.

A second-degree burn, that has blisters and superficial damage to the outer layer of skin, but is not very large, is treated in the same way as a first degree burn. However, it is important to watch closely for any indication of breaking blisters or infection and to get prompt medical treatment.

A third-degree burn, which causes blistering and damages the deeper layers of the skin, is a serious injury that requires immediate medical treatment, particularly on lymphedema-affected tissues.

Now you know my behind the scenes professional secrets for wound care; sorry no other recipes included here.

Remy

Dreaded Jock Itch

"If you start to get a rash, act immediately and you can clear it up very quickly."

Editors' Note: We just had to include this real-life advice about a seldom-discussed but very important topic that affects women as well as men. Learn how one woman deals with the problem.

I live in North Carolina and upon retirement turned into a gardener (to my total surprise). All those stories you have heard about North Carolina summer heat and humidity are true, and then some. Add on Class Four Plus compression stockings and you have the perfect environment for jock itch. Yeow! (Note: The medical term for jock itch is *tinea cruris*. It is a fungal infection very similar to athlete's foot except that it occurs in the genital area.)

Of course, the most sensible way to avoid jock itch is to stay inside and avoid sweating. Scrap that idea; I'm going to be out in that garden. Sensible Plan B is to change out of the sweating compression stockings as soon as they become wet. Well, that would be in five minutes. Besides, it takes 20 minutes to get out of clammy stockings, dry off, and put on a new pair. And that assumes you have a second pair that's not all worn out to put on.

This leaves us with Plan C. C is for compromise. I wear underpants that wick away moisture to some degree. This year I am also trying incontinence pads. (At my age I wear them not just for jock itch!). They do a great job of wicking away moisture in general. Since we've only have about a dozen 80 degree days so far (hey, it's only April), I haven't given the pads the full test yet, put I am very hopeful.

But, in spite of all precautions, you might get jock itch. It really really hurts! That's the bad news. The good news is that it responds extremely quickly to medication. I use an over-the-counter absorbent powder as soon as I come in from the garden. My dermatologist has prescribed two ointments to use if the rash does appear. These ointments work miracles overnight. So the message is, if you start to get a rash act immediately and you can clear it up very quickly.

Avid Gardener

Treating a Child with Lymphedema

"Treating a child with lymphedema can be challenging and well worth the effort!"

Editors' Note: When faced first with a five year old and then a ten month old, both requiring manual lymph drainage and compression, Judith Sedlak knew she had a challenge on her hands.

Here are some marvelous tips that will be helpful to any therapist treating a child with lymphedema and to every parent of a child with lymphedema.

Getting children to participate in physical therapy is a challenge. It requires finding a balance between fun and work, and that is sometimes difficult!

Treating a child with lymphedema has the special challenges of getting them to sit still for manual lymph drainage or convincing them to keep their compression wrapping on. Such a challenge is well worth the effort.

My first child with lymphedema was only five years old when he came to me. How would I ever get him to lie still for me? How would I ever convince him to keep his leg wrapped in bulky compression wrapping while playing with his friends at school?

The second child I saw was only 10 months old. How would I ever get an active baby who was just learning to crawl to sit still during treatment?

Here are some tricks that have worked for me:

- Use hand held video games—even inexpensive ones—that can be played with in any position!

- Play word games—think of those games we have all played on long road trips—"I went to the store and bought...," "Geography" (name a location, and the next person names one that starts with the last letter of yours), "I spy," "I am thinking of a word that starts with the letter... (Or the sound...)

- Have your child hold a book for you to read out loud—or, have your child practice reading to you. This even works for non-readers—have them "tell" you the story from the pictures.

- Practice math facts—flash cards are helpful!

- Videos, DVD's, favorite TV shows help quiet the restless child!

- Make a "lymphedema box" with favorite toys, books, videos that are used only when you are doing CDT. Let the child pick out what they want to play with. Rotate the toys if your child is getting bored.

- With younger children set yourself up in a confined space—put pillows around you to define the space or work in a small corner. Allow the child some opportunity to move around. If it is an arm that's involved, make sure to allow some time for those little fingers to play with toys!

- Have someone else entertain the child while you work—this is especially helpful for younger children and when you aren't confident in what you are doing.

- Write out the steps of CDT or take pictures of each step—have your child keep track of what step you are on, tell you what comes next, etc.

- Explain to the child what you are doing and why—in their terms. Have them help you—they can help rub lotion on, tear pieces of tape for the bandages and even help wrap—even if it is just the end of the last bandage. This helps empower the child and teaches them how they can take care of their lymphedema.

- Allow the child to put stickers on their bandages when their arm or leg is all wrapped.

- If you take measurements, share them with your child—show them the progress they are making by wearing their bandages (and of course show them the change that happens if they don't!). If done as a graph, even a young child can see that the line is going down as their arm/leg is getting smaller.

- Use child-friendly terms: a garment can be a "special sock" or a "magic glove."

- Above all, be patient and do what you can! Anything is better than nothing!

Judith Sedlak, PT, CLT

Editors' Note: Ruthi provided some additional tips as part of her review.

Some suggestions, tips from my personal experience with treating children:

- When you take circumference measurements, you can give the child also a measuring tape. Let him measure the other leg or a doll's leg.

- Let the child roll the bandages.

- For abdominal breathing, give the child soap bubbles to blow and tell them "…blow very slowly, so the bubble will get bigger and bigger." It really helps and is fun.

Ruthi Peleg, BPt, BS, CLT

Answering Questions about Bandages or Compression Garments

"My, that looks interesting."

Editors' Note: What do you think of Marcene's responses? What do you say?

What other people with lymphedema ask me most frequently is, "How do you handle questions about your bandages or compression garment?" I'm happy to share the answers that work well for me.

Just last week in the gym dressing room when I was putting on my sleeve, a lady said, "My, that looks interesting, tell me about it." I thought that was such a polite way to inquire about my sleeve.

With adults, I reply, "It is a condition caused by my cancer treatment and it is called lymphedema. I wear these bandages or sleeve to keep my arm from swelling. It does a good job and I am well now."

If they want more information, then I tell them more about it. Often they know someone with a swollen limb. I always encourage them to tell their acquaintance that it is treatable and to seek treatment.

When young children ask, I reply: "I was sick and the treatment makes my arm swell up. This sleeve keeps my arm from swelling and I am all better now." Usually that is all they want to know.

I hope this may help someone feel more at ease with their lymphedema treatment.

Marcene Johansson

I Talk About Lymphedema

"I'm helping to grease the skids toward the day when lymphedema will no longer be a silent epidemic."

Editors' Note: Mary Pat shares how she takes every chance to educate others about lymphedema.

Whenever I can, to whomever I can, I believe in talking about my lymphedema. So many people know nothing about it and this makes it harder for those of us who have it. I don't go up to strangers on the street and start running off at the mouth or anything, but whenever I get a question that leads me to lymphedema, I talk as openly as I can about it.

Every time I educate someone just a little bit about lymphedema I feel like I'm helping to grease the skids toward the day when lymphedema will no longer be a silent epidemic.

Mary Pat B.

Treating Infections

"No MLD or compression while the affected area is hot, red and painful."

Editors' Note: No matter how careful you are, there are times when an arm or leg affected by lymphedema becomes infected. We've included guidelines for recognizing an infection in the Appendix, see page 209.

Here are Marcene's suggestions. After you start treating an infection, check with your therapist for guidelines on when you can safely resume treatment, self-massage, and compression.

My big problem is infections. I have from 6-8 infections a year no matter how careful I am. Sometimes it is a small wound; sometimes I just do not know the cause. I do know that starting antibiotics quickly is essential.

The sooner the antibiotics start, the sooner the infection will go away and I can again work at getting the swelling down. In the meantime, the guideline is no MLD or compression while the affected area is hot, red, painful, or still showing signs of infection.

At all times I try hard to protect my arm against any injury that might cause yet another infection, but sometimes it happens.

Marcene Johansson

Editors' Note: Here are some additional tips for managing this common problem:

- Ask your physician for a stand-by antibiotic prescription with instructions on when to start taking the medication for skin infection, how to take the medication, and how long to continue taking the medication.

- Have this prescription filled even if you don't have an infection. If you develop an infection and you can't reach your doctor, start taking the antibiotic as instructed.

- Any time you use your stand-by antibiotics, be sure to tell your doctor right away, ask for another stand-by antibiotic prescription, and get that prescription filled.

- Be sure and tell your doctor about all your infections, including minor ones. Your doctor may prescribe preventative antibiotics if you are having frequent infections.

- Keep your skin well moisturized. This helps it to better withstand minor bumps and scrapes.

- If you are going to be in the sun, always wear good sunscreen and reapply it as needed.

- Wear gloves for gardening, housework, or any task that might cause a break in the skin. Long sleeves and insect repellent help too.

- If you have even a minor scrape or break in the skin, treat the wound and apply antibiotic ointment.

- If an insect bites you on the affected tissue, clean the area of the bite and apply antibiotic ointment.

- Anytime you have an injury, no matter how minor, check it at least once a day for signs of infection.

- Review with your doctor whether you might have any other health issues that could contribute to developing infections.

- Review your treatment regimen with your lymphedema therapist to determine if there are changes in your routine that might reduce the number of infections.

Editors' Note: Do you have standby antibiotics (and are they current?), or an up-to-date prescription for antibiotics? Do you know when to start the antibiotic and when to call your doctor or other treating professional? If you don't, put these questions on your list for your next doctor's visit.

Chapter **7**

Self-Care Tips

Here are even more creative, practical tips. These suggestions come from people just like you who know what it is like living day after day with lymphedema, or from professionals who treat lymphedema.

We learned a lot from the contributors who so generously shared practical advice and suggestions. We hope you will too.

Caution: Of course, always check with your lymphedema therapist or health care professional before changing your routine based on something you read or hear.

We don't give medical advice and what works for one person may not work for someone else. But we encourage you to let others' experiences lead to creative ideas that work for you.

Tips from Beth

"Before and after pictures show improvement and document progress!"

Editors' Note: Beth Shapiro, MS, OTR/L-CLT shares her suggestions about common lymphedema issues.

Caution: Remember that everyone is different. With all health-related advice throughout the book, we advise you to check with your health care team first before changing what you do.

- Mr. Clean brand orange latex gloves are helpful to don and doff compression garments. Using the gloves helps to prevent rips in the garment. Also the grip on the palm and fingers assists the garment in sliding on and off the limb.

- Stay well hydrated particularly in hot weather. This means drinking lots of cool water and avoiding excessive caffeine or alcohol which act as diuretics.

- If you are salt-sensitive, you may find it best to avoid eating more than 2,500 mg of salt a day. Some health conditions, such as high blood pressure, may require a more restricted sodium intake. Talk to your physician.

- Boudreaux's Butt Paste, which is marketed primarily for use in treating diaper rash, is also considered by many to be an effective healer of almost everything including blisters and superficial wounds. For more details, visit the Boudreaux's Butt Paste web site (www.buttpaste.com).

- A thin layer of Aquaphor ointment placed on gauze, or other covering material, is helpful in treating wounds. This ointment prevents the gauze from sticking to the wound when the dressing is changed. *Aquaphor Healing Ointment* is a Eucerin product described as being beneficial by protecting dry, cracked or irritated skin and helping to enhance the natural healing process to restore smooth, healthy skin.

- I caution my clients against allowing deep tissue massage to be performed on lymphedema-affected tissues! Deep tissue work, performed inappropriately, can worsen lymphedema.

- An Aquashield is a completely watertight cover that enables you to shower and bathe normally while wearing a compression garment or bandages. Commonly known as a waterproof cast cover, this shield creates a tight seal over the bandages. Because this is tight, I recommend that you limit the time wearing it to taking a quick shower or bath!

- Take before and after pictures (and record the date and time). These show changes and document progress!

Beth (Elizabeth) Shapiro, MS, OTR/L, CLT

Self-Massage in the Morning

"The alarm goes off in the morning and I hit the snooze button."

Editors' Note: We are always happy to find a reason to spend a few more minutes in bed before getting up to face the day. This is Mary Pat's suggestion for building self-massage into a daily routine.

I've made self-massage easier for myself by doing it first thing in the morning. The alarm goes off in the morning and I hit snooze. Then I do self-massage until it goes off again.

This gets the self-massage done for the morning, and it makes it perfectly legitimate for me to wait an extra 10 minutes before I get off the bed.

Mary Pat B.

Editors' Note: Ruthi added this advice as part of her manuscript review:

I advise my patients to choose the right/proper time for self-massage. I suggest a time when you are alone, not under stress to take care of the family, or in a hurry to get to work in the morning. Each person has his/her own schedule and can find the perfect time.

For a parent who has to get the children out for school on time, the mornings may not be right. Think about a time that is convenient for you, when you know this time is just for you, without interruptions. You can put on nice music or a talk show on TV while massaging, exercising.

Ruthi Peleg, BPt, BS, CLT

Self-Care and Meditation

"The key for me has been to turn challenges into opportunities for growth—to spin straw into gold."

Editors' Note: Read this story of one man's spiritual growth in response to lymphedema and how he uses his daily care time for reflection.

Instead of reporting a straight chronology of my experiences with lymphedema, which affects my leg, I discovered that my story is better suited to describing how it has influenced the areas of my life. I'm focusing here on the spiritual aspects.

Lymphedema has been something of a blow to my male ego, but has contributed to a greater sense of humility. I feel now that I carry a wound, a weakness, and this awareness can be of considerable value in relating to others with greater vulnerability and empathy.

Although initially I was inclined to hide the lymphedema, I am now much more open about it, and am not shy about doing some minor self-massage when I am with others. The clear sense of my physical imperfection, and the visibility of this, has led to a greater sense of compassion not only as a concept, but as a way of being.

My inclination toward mysticism and different models of interaction with the divine has also been energized. The care required for my lymphedema has allowed me to extend and solidify some of the daily practices of prayer, meditation, and bodily awareness that were already part of my routine.

When I realized that I would need to spend time each morning and evening tending to my leg, I resolved to make the best use of this time by directing it toward structured spiritual practice.

There are types of bodily awareness exercises, meditation, and prayer that accompany each part of my exercise and massage regimen. This combining of physical self-care with spiritual attention has deepened my spiritual practice and has increased my level of reflectiveness and presence.

I am aware that the state of my leg may change and present me with new challenges. I am aware, also, that there may surface aspects of my response to the condition that will require some reorientation. I am intent, however, on responding to any changes or discoveries as positively as I can, recognizing what I can change and what I cannot change.

I recall the serenity prayer: asking to have the serenity to accept the things one cannot change, the courage to change the things one can, and the wisdom to know the difference. I think that what has been the key for me in my lymphedema story has been to balance acceptance with active agency and, whenever I can see how, to turn challenges into opportunities for growth— to spin straw into gold.

Brent

Garment Donning Suggestion

"Donning Garments can be difficult!"

Editors' Note: Getting compression garments on and off can be a tiresome, time-consuming, frustrating process! Renee shares her tips.

Donning of garments, especially lower leg stockings can be difficult. As a fitter, I find people are able to better don their garment using the special rubber fitting gloves (not the regular Playtex gloves found in the supermarket) because the traction pads on the palm of the glove help move the material up the leg, rather than pulling on the band and overstretching the garment.

Using a small amount of ALPS Fitting Lotion on the heel also helps the garment slip up well. This lotion, distributed by Juzo, is silicone based, hypoallergenic, and contains no perfumes or dyes.

Renee Romero, RN, CLT-LANA

Editors' Note: as part of his review Bob Weiss offered some additional suggestions:

We use the Jobst Easy Slide aid that makes donning a compression sleeve a breeze.

A bandage roller—the best $13.00 dollar investment I ever made.

Robert Weiss, MS

Wrapping as Family Time

"You have to control the lymphedema, not let it control you."

Editors' Note: Susan shares a marvelous example of building lymphedema self-care into ongoing family life.

I was diagnosed with primary lymphedema when I was 36 years old. I have it mainly in my left leg. The one thing I would stress is maintenance. You can not let it go. I wrap my legs religiously (with a night off here and there) and wear compression hosiery or CircAid everyday.

My husband helps me roll my wrapping garments while we are relaxing in front of the TV. I also wrap my legs with our two kids (ages 9 and 6) and my husband while we are watching TV together. My younger son said to me once, *"Mom, does everyone's mom wrap their legs?"*

For swimming, I wear a Tankini top with swim pants to cover my legs. If I didn't do that, my legs would look like elephant trunks.

You have to control the lymphedema, not let it control you. I am a very active 40 year-old and I exercise 4 or 5 days a week. Most importantly, I don't let lymphedema stop me from doing anything.

Susan Klapper

Increased Comfort during Long Meetings

"If lymphedema affects your legs, there is a kind of self-massage that is useful when you have to sit for a long time."

Editors' Note: Brent shares a specific tip for those with lower extremity lymphedema.

If lymphedema affects your legs, here is a kind of self-massage that is useful and can be done in many situations such as sitting in movie theatres, through long meetings, as a passenger on a long car trip, over dinner, or on airplane flights.

I massage the Achilles tendon area of the affected leg by using some ankle pumping (moving the foot up and down). This moves the muscles that in turn stimulate the lymph drainage and allows me to sit more comfortably for extended periods of time.

Brent

Heavy Traffic and Lymphedema Exercises

"Traffic jams are a perfect place for doing some self-care exercises."

Editors' Note: We are so impressed by the creativity shown by our contributors in finding ways to work self-massage into their daily lives. Here are Emily's suggestions.

I can do quite a few of my exercises while I'm commuting. Red lights and traffic jams are perfect for shoulder rolls, flexing arms, squeezing hands, and such. They are also great for clearing nodes.

I'm already stuck in the car, so the self-care doesn't take any extra time out of my life. Just remember to keep an eye on traffic to be ready to move when it does!

Sometimes I do these things while I'm on the phone too. It's a good way for me to kill two birds with one stone.

Emily P. Bees

Editors' Note: Ruthi added these suggestions in her review of the manuscript:

- You can perform your self-massage in the shower; it is easier with soap and a sponge.

- Exercise in front of the TV.

- When you don't have enough time to perform the whole self-massage, instead of not doing it at all, just massage the central parts (lymph node clearing, breathing), then put on the compression garment (morning) or the bandages (night).

Ruthi Peleg, BPt, BS, CLT

When the Top of Your Hand Swells

"My biggest problem is still the swelling in the back of my hand."

Editors' Note: Special thanks to Marci Johansson for submitting this tip for Melba who explained, "I still do not do e-mail (yet)!"

I am a 35-year survivor of cancer and lymphedema. My arm is as large as it was 15 years ago before lymphedema treatment was available, but now it is maintained at that size. My biggest problem is still the swelling in the back of my hand.

Here is my tip for managing this. When the top of your hands swells, sit on it. I tuck my hand under my bottom while watching TV or riding in the car and it helps to bring the swelling down.

Successful Night Compression

"The best choice of night compression is wrapping with short stretch bandages!"

Editors' Note: David Adcock, a certified lymphedema therapist and physical therapist, shares lessons from his experience.

As a lymphedema therapist, one of my major challenges is to convince patients to wear compression at night. Nighttime compression is a must because at night, when they are not active, most patients gain excess fluid.

The best choice for night compression is wrapping with short-stretch bandages. However, wrapping presents a variety of challenges: it can be tedious and time consuming, and many individuals are unable to self-wrap yet have no one to assist them.

My experience is that when clients tire of this routine, they cease doing it. However without nightly compression, the volume of the affected limb progressively increases.

There are effective options for solving this challenge. These include teaching techniques that makes it easier to apply the short stretch bandages. Once the client has mastered the skill, and it has become part of the daily routine, it is no longer a "big deal" to wrap.

Depending on the situation, I have found that some clients do better with other products to replace bandaging. Some of these options include: JoViPak garments (www.jovipak.com); Reid Sleeve, Opera, or Contour Plus from Peninsula Medical Supply (www.lymphedema.com); CircAid (www.lymphedema.biz), and Farrow Wrap (www.farrowmedical.com).

All of these products are more expensive than wrapping with bandages. And for the majority of individuals who do not have insurance that will cover these costs, the expense is prohibitive. At this point creativity becomes necessary.

When a claim for one of these garments is denied, providing full information and documented outcomes to the third party payer can sometimes enable approval. This issue should be resolved before ordering a garment for a client who cannot pay for it without insurance coverage.

There are philanthropic sources that will assist in providing financial aid. For example some hospitals have special funds to meet these needs. Contact a social worker at the hospital to see if such aid is available. (See the list of organizations in the Appendix.)

Another source of help is to contact the manufacturers these garments; often they have excess inventory that they will donate.

Some support groups hold fund raising events to help with the cost of such garments. (See Chapter 9 for information on support groups.)

Lymphedema can be managed. Management of lymphedema can become very doable. Speak with your lymphedema therapist to find your best option.

David Adcock, PT, CLT

Beating the Heat

"My belief is you control your lymphedema; it does not control your life."

Editors' Note: Marcene has arm lymphedema after breast cancer treatment. She and some of her Lymph Notes friends who have lymphedema affecting their legs share their tips on ways to "beat the heat" and stay cool in hot weather.

- I use a piece of cardboard covered with aluminum foil to keep the sun off my arm when riding in the car.

- When my arm and chest become overheated, I use a bag of frozen peas to cool it down. I move the bag over my chest and sleeve more in the direction of the lymph flow. Never leave it in one place, but keep it moving slowly. Start with the chest and back area first after your breathing exercises.

- *Suggestion from a friend*: I use a "Cool Gel-Pak" that lives in my freezer. I wrap it in several layers of a towel, so it isn't too cold against the skin. When I get cool, and the Gel-Pak gets warm, it goes back in the freezer and I go about my day.

- I have found the best way to cool your lymphedema down is a cool shower, but unfortunately that is not always an option.

- *Suggestion from a friend*: Another great solution is to get into the swimming pool of cool water. Go deep enough to cover the base of your skull. This cools your body core temperature and feels really great! This is also a good time to do self-massage and some exercises.

- **Here is an idea that I tried that did NOT work!** I squirted water on my sleeve to cool down by evaporation. This was cooling but I developed an infection that I think may have been caused by doing it.

- *Suggestion from a friend*: I keep my knit compression sleeve in the refrigerator overnight wrapped in a plastic bag so it won't get damp. This way I begin my day with a cooler garment.

- I always carry my water bottle with me. Sometimes I use an insulated bottle. Other times I use a plastic bottle that is only partway filled. I put it in the freezer until I'm ready to go out and, as it thaws, it provides me with a supply of pleasantly cool water. With the cap on tight, rubbing that cold bottle against the back of my neck helps to cool my core body temperature as well.

- *Suggestion from a friend*: I think that long roomy skirts are cooler than shorts. They allow air circulation and when you sit down you don't have to keep your legs together, so they sweat less.

Good luck in the heat and humidity. My belief is you control your lymphedema; it does not control your life.

Marcene Johansson and friends

Chapter **8**

Humor Helps

Editors' Note: Many of our contributors mentioned the importance of humor in coping with the demands of lymphedema. Here are some contributors who address it directly or who demonstrate how they use humor themselves. Enjoy!

My Wrapping Saga

"Wrap. Oops. Re-roll. Wrap. Ooops. Tape. Yes!"

Editors' Note: Jackie uses humor to present a dilemma with which you may be very familiar. As she recounts her wrapping saga, the fire-safety phrase "stop, drop, and roll" takes on a whole new meaning!

For your enjoyment: Time: 7:38 am

Put the undersleeve on, get all the wrinkles out, make sure the thumb holes are in the right place.

Wrap the foam.

Foam doesn't go up the arm high enough. Unwrap, re-roll, Re-wrap.

Realize I should have wrapped the fingers first. Unwrap foam, re-roll.

Wrap fingers.

Oops, dropped the roll. Re-roll, continue wrapping.

Wrap with first bandage. Good job. Oops forgot to get the tape ready. No problem. Tape. Yes!

Fold the undersleeve over the bandage. Hmmmmmmm. Not enough undersleeve. Something is wrong at the fingers. Thumb won't go into second hole on undersleeve. Ooops. Forgot to wrap the foam. Unwrap bandage. Re-roll.

Wrap foam. Oops. Not far enough. Unwrap, re-roll, re-wrap.

Fold undersleeve over foam at hand. Thumb hole a little tight, but that's okay.

Next bandage. Wrap. Wrap. Drop the roll. Re-roll. Wrap. Wrap. Tape.

Next bandage. Wrap. Wrap. Wrap. Tape. Tape. Tape.

Time: 8:25 am: Sigh. Tomorrow will be better.

Update: Down to 20 Minutes

As a matter of fact, this morning I got the deed done in 20 minutes! I'm going to try to beat that record, however, because I'm going to London soon with friends. I don't want to hold everyone up in the morning while I wrap. So I'm shooting for 10 minutes. I think I can. I think I can!

Jackie Doss

One of your editors was inspired to write new words to the children's song "Row, Row, Row Your Boat" for this occasion:
Roll, roll, roll your bandage; Gently 'round the limb;
Wrap, wrap, wrap and tape; 'Til you get it trim.

Advantages of Bilateral Lower Extremity Lymphedema

"Here is my list of advantages. What would you add to it?"

Editors' Note: Dixie uses her delightful sense of humor to find a bright side, or at least a smile, out of living with bilateral lower extremity lymphedema.

Finding anything advantageous about having bilateral lower extremity lymphedema is a challenge for even the most optimistic among us; however, it is achievable. Here is my list of advantages. What would you add to it?

- Bilateral lower extremity lymphedema is good for your back. Because of the bandages, you don't have to sleep with a pillow between your knees to keep that lower back straight. Cool!

- You save money because you don't have to buy slippers. What's the point of slippers? You need to keep your feet in lace-up shoes while you have your garments on during the day. When you switch to Jovi padded leggings or bandages in the evening, you can't fit slippers over them. What a saving over the years!

- You save even more money because you don't have to bother buying pantyhose. I don't know about you, but I can run a pair of pantyhose just by looking at them. Here is another item that can be removed from the budget!

- You never have to worry about a Halloween costume. You can alternate between going as the Mummy and the Michelin Man.

- You might get a pity upgrade on an airline. Since they get too uncomfortable because you can't move around, you can't wear compression stockings on long flights. So you wear your Jovi padded stockings and cast boots. The key to the upgrade is <u>not</u> to look pitiful and <u>not</u> to ask for an upgrade. Just clump on through the endless lines, dragging your luggage behind you. Soldier on, be brave. You might find yourself in first class!!!

Dixie Spiegel

Farewell to the Underwire Bra

"Sorry, can't even look at 'em."

Editors' Note: Sometimes you're happy to say farewell to something because of lymphedema! Here is an example from Anonymous.

One good thing that came out of lymphedema was being told I should never wear an underwire bra again! Sorry, can't even look at 'em, medical orders you know. Actually it was fun tossing out these old instruments of torture.

Anonymous

Chapter 9

Support Groups

Editors' Note: These stories illustrate the powerful impact of support. We have stories about online resources, resources for Native Americans, informal support networks, stories from successful groups, and tips on organizing a support group.

Sharing knowledge about lymphedema not only helps others, it may even make you happier! The latest research on happiness finds that sustained happiness comes from leading an engaged, meaningful life. Teaching and mentoring others clarifies and deepens your understanding. It engages your mind and your spirit.

To find a support group, check the directory under Lymphedema Resources on Lymph Notes (www.LymphNotes.com). Lymphedema treatment centers and breast care centers will have information on local support groups. Many support groups welcome all types of lymphedema even if the group is breast cancer oriented.

Online Friends

"It feels so good to know that I am not alone with this condition."

Editors' Note: This post to the LymphNotes Forums highlights the emotional impact of lymphedema and how many people with lymphedema feel isolated. It beautifully expresses how helpful online support can be to someone with lymphedema. Online Forums have the advantage of being available anywhere there is an Internet connection and any time.

We hope you find sources of support in your own life, and that you find ways to offer support and help to others.

My name is Melanie. I'm 33 and I've had lymphedema since I was a teenager. It's frustrating and overwhelming at times. I never met anyone else who has this condition. I had to cope with high school, and college, and going on job interviews, all on my own. It has felt so lonely.

I don't mean to complain. I learned to manage the swelling and how to answer rude questions about my garments and bandages. I even found a wonderful man who loves me despite the lymphedema. We've been married for 10 years now and we have two bright, beautiful children. I know I'm really lucky.

But in all my travels (and I've traveled quite a bit!), I never saw one other person wearing a compression garment or with their leg wrapped. It wasn't until I found this website and these forums that I realized there are a lot of other folks out there facing the same problems I do. It feels so good to know that I am not alone with this condition. At last I have friends I can "talk" to about my feelings, even if we never meet in person.

It means a lot to me to have "friends" who know what it's like to cope with wrapping in hot weather or to try to look stylish with swollen legs. The bandages can make it hard to get around. And they can feel so confining. Sometimes I get pretty down. There are so many emotions it's hard to express.

I'm so glad I found other people to talk to about lymphedema who share my experience. I really appreciate your compassion and support. And it's amazing how much I have learned. I wish I could say a personal "thank you" to each of you. I can't express how much you have helped me. I think we all draw strength from one another. It is so wonderful!

Melanie

Native American Healing Ceremonies

"There is much we can learn about recognizing and maintaining spiritual balance."

Editors' Note: Spiritual and religious beliefs can be a tremendous source of support. We thank Laurie for passing on to our readers this unusual support resource for Native Americans. Where do you turn to for support?

The Native American Cancer Research website (www.natamcancer.org) includes a lymphedema branch designed to help Native Americans learn how to live with their lymphedema. This site provides excellent information as told in the ancient native tradition of stories combined with the modern medium of video.

The spiritual needs of the patient are recognized and instructions are included on the ways in which traditional healing ceremonies can be modified so that individuals with lymphedema can take part while avoiding the risk of developing an infection due to a break in the skin.

Although specifically designed to help Native Americans, there is much that all of us can learn from this website—perhaps most importantly—the importance of recognizing and maintaining spiritual balance as a means of moving toward improved health.

Laurie Feest, OTR, CHT, LLCC

We Share and Talk as We Wait

"These afternoons help each of us."

Editors' Note: Formal support groups are not the only way to give and receive support. Here Marcene gives a wonderful example of turning what is an irritation for most of us (sitting in the waiting room) into a source of mutual comfort, support, and education.

Reaching out to others can happen anywhere!

Each month my therapists have an afternoon when patients can come in for a check-up to see how well their lymphedema is maintained. On these afternoons, I encourage the patients to talk together as we wait our turn.

It has turned out to be a very important support group for many of us. I am always amazed at how fearful lymphedema patients are, even when they are doing very well.

I think these afternoons help each of us feel so much better about living with lymphedema.

Marcene Johansson

The WVLN Support Group in Action

"On a scale of 1 to 10 for good support group meetings, I'd say that last night's was 110."

Editors' Note: Tracy Novak reports on a recent meeting of the West Virginia Lymphedema Network (WVLN), a volunteer organization based in Morgantown. The support group maintains a website (www.wvlymph.org) and meets quarterly.

Our support group met last evening. I don't want to brag or anything but the meeting was great with 15 people attending. This included two certified therapists, one Occupational Therapy (OT) student, four new people and the rest were our "old timers." Three people drove all the way from Maryland to West Virginia to attend.

The meeting was extremely dynamic. One person, who has primary lymph-edema of the leg, shared with the group new information and contacts from a primary lymphedema meeting she had attended in Pittsburgh.

The new people expressed their fears and concerns and the whole group was a fountain of good advice for them. Our normal "Caring and Sharing" time is 30 minutes, but last night it was 90 minutes and could easily have gone another hour.

There was a lot of talk about infections. Three from the group experience infections on a regular basis, which I think is a big number considering there were only 12 patients at the meeting (the others are medical professionals).

The OT student has been doing research on lymphedema insurance issues. She has also created a DVD containing information plus bandaging and exercise demos. We're going to make copies and distribute them free to the group. The bandaging demo is particularly valuable.

Beth, our speaker on exercises, presented the new research about exercise and lymphedema. Then she provided handouts and we all practiced the ex-ercises with her.

After our exercises, we shared a cake in Beth's honor. At this moment Beth was the most loved and hated person in the room. Loved because she means so much to us and was one of the founding directors of our support group. Hated, not really, because she is leaving to move to Ecuador with her husband where they will live and travel for a year. She's a wonderful person and she will be dearly missed.

On a scale of 1 to 10 for good support group meetings, I'd say that last night's was 110 (except for Beth's leaving). At the end of the meeting, people didn't want to leave and stayed and continued to talk in little groups.

Reported by Tracy Novak

"Sharing our joys and concerns with each other provides an outlet that we don't have anywhere else."

"Support group meetings reenergize me!"

Editors' Note: Group members express their opinions of the benefits of attending an ongoing, in-person support group.

- The support group provides a valuable "community" for you in which others understand where you are coming from. It is a wonderful forum to exchange ideas and to lean the most you can about managing lymphedema.

- Hearing about all the latest treatment and new ideas about lymphedema; my favorite meetings are the ones in which a specialist in some area of lymphedema presents to us. You also see all of your friends.

- I found it helpful to hear how others have dealt with the problems I am experiencing. The best was that people are doing research on their own and sharing info, websites, etc. with the rest of us.

- Support group meetings reenergize me to do the things that I need to do to manage my lymphedema. Without these meetings, I would be a very poor patient instead of the smiling compliant patient that I am!

- The caring and sharing are the most important part of the meetings for me. Sharing our joys and concerns with each other provides an outlet that we don't have anywhere else.

The Lymphedema Education and Resource Group

"We are dedicated to helping each other to cope with, and manage, this life-changing condition."

Editors' Note: After Jayah recounted her adventures with lymphedema to her radiation oncologist (see page 12) she was referred to the woman who coordinated breast cancer care of for the hospital. As a result, Jayah helped form the Lymphedema Education and Resource Group.

The motto of our group is, *"Timely intervention is critical for managing lymphedema. We are dedicated to helping each other cope with, and manage, this life-changing condition."*

Meetings are free and anyone is invited to attend. We meet on the third Wednesday of every month in the Breast Health Center of the California Pacific Medical Center.

Meetings include an educational presentation, plus time for questions and practical techniques for understanding and managing lymphedema to help the members understand, manage and prevent lymphedema.

More information is available on the Adventure Buddies website (www.adventurebuddies.net).

Jayah Faye Paley

We Feel Honored to Share our Knowledge

"It is our pleasure to improve understanding by providing the community with education."

Editors' Note: Nancy, a certified lymphedema therapist, talks about how she reaches out to support and educate others.

I am one of the lymphedema therapists at the Lehigh Valley Hospital and Health Network in Lehigh Valley, Pennsylvania. We feel honored to be able to share our knowledge and experience with the local community. When speaking to each community group our topic is personalized to meet their particular needs.

In general, our themes include lymphedema education, treatment options, risk reduction, and exercise. These are all framed with compassion and we often speak to cancer and lymphedema support groups.

Bimonthly we speak to individuals who will soon be having breast cancer surgery. Our goal is to educate these patients and to allay their fears about lymphedema. We also include exercises for them before and after surgery.

We regularly speak at ongoing classes for cancer survivors at a local Wellness Community Center and offer concurrent educational sessions as part of the hospital's one day Breast Cancer Survivor's Workshop.

Since burn patients share many of the difficulties faced by those with lymphedema, we also participate in the semiannual two-day *"Beyond the Burn"* program for recovering burn patients and their families.

Our latest initiative is collaborating with the Weight Management Center in an effort to serve overweight individuals who also have lymphedema.

There is a lack of public knowledge about lymphedema, risk reduction, and treatment. It is our pleasure to improve their understanding by providing the community with education and therapeutic intervention.

Nancy Kinzli, MS, ORT/L, CLT-LANA

Saved by Community Outreach

"If it had not been for this lecture, I would not know what to do!"

Editors' Note: We love being able to follow Nancy's story with Lorelei's. Read about the impact of outreach. How did you first learn about lymphedema? Have you helped others learn about it?

I first heard about lymphedema at a Luci Curci Cancer Center lecture about a month ago. Before this meeting, I had no idea that I was supposed to take precautions while flying, exercising, or doing every day things. If it were not for this lecture, I would not know what to do.

Danielle Meglio, from Eisenhower Medical Center in Palm Desert California, discussed preventive care and the importance of massage therapy. I have been going three times a week for four weeks and have learned how to do the lymph massage on myself. Danielle sees a lot of women from this lecture. Unfortunately, she only presents this program once a year but I am trying to convince her to have it at least twice a year.

Lorelei Foss

Spreading Our Wings

"The goal of this event was to raise money for financial aid to those with lymphedema who cannot afford treatment essentials."

Editors' Note: Finally, here is Michelle's recipe for doing good and having fun. It sounds great to us!

The "Spreading Our Wings Fashion Show and Champagne Luncheon" was a successful fund raising event organized by the members of the Lymphedema Support Group working in cooperation with the Dominican Lymphedema Clinic, the Dominican Hospital and the Katz Cancer Resource Center in Santa Cruz County, California.

The goal of this event was to raise money for a fund that provides financial aid to those with lymphedema who cannot afford treatment essentials such as compression garments and bandages that are not covered by medical insurance.

A second goal of the event was to help those with lymphedema feel better about their self-image. This goal was met by the fashion show using lymphedema clients as models.

The event was sold out with 200 people attending. As a fundraiser it was highly successful by raising nearly $15,000 for the Lymphedema Patient Support Fund at Dominican Hospital Foundation. Best of all, it was fun, we had a good time working together, and the models were inspiring.

Michelle Shippen

Editors' Postscript: This example shared by Michelle is only one of many groups who participate in fund-raising, outreach, and philanthropy.

Supporting Each Other in a Lifestyle Change

"We are leading productive lives in spite of having, and dealing with, lymphedema."

Editors' Note: Suzi talks about how powerful it is to have support, encouragement, and good role models when dealing with lymphedema. Yes, you have to deal with lymphedema; and "life goes on."

One way we help each other in our support group is to encourage compliance with the known lymphedema therapies.

Newcomers in particular are really shocked that they might have to bandage for an extended period of time or are told that they will have to do self-massage and have to wear a compression garment probably for the rest of their life.

This is a terrible lifestyle change for many. They resist it. They don't want to do it. Neither did I, in fact, I hated it! However, these individuals need to be convinced that early compliance should keep their lymphedema from worsening.

The members of the group are able to demonstrate to them that we have been doing this for years and we are not freaks. We are living really normal and productive happy lives. Our sex lives are not destroyed. We have jobs. We are active women. And life goes on.

Newcomers are encouraged when they realize that we are a group of attractive, educated, and productive women and men who are leading productive lives in spite of having, and dealing with, lymphedema.

Suzi Beatie

Starting and Maintaining a Support Group

"We respect privacy. What is said in the group stays in the group."

Editors' Note: The preceding stories talked about the benefit of informal and online support. Are you feeling inspired to join or start a support group?

Suzi shares her tips on starting and maintaining a successful support group. Read on!

We started the Marin Lymphedema Information & Support Group in 2000. It seems like yesterday, but it's been seven years now. We started accidentally in a way. There was a need and another woman and I just filled it. We had neither experience nor other support group involvement. But there were women who needed help and had no where to turn, so sometimes you just need to open up your heart and be there. Here are some of the factors we have discovered to be important in successfully starting and running a support group:

- **An umbrella helps.** We operate under the "umbrella" of our local hospital. This is beneficial because they provide a meeting room and they advertise our meetings in the hospital newsletters. This is a great way to reach potential new members.

- **Planners.** It works better when more than one person is starting a new support group. These individuals need to work together and be responsible for scheduling and planning meetings. To avoid burnout, it is best to rotate these roles. Being part of this role is also an excellent way to get people truly involved in the group.

- **Know your audience.** When making plans, it is important to recognize and meet the needs of your group with programs that match the interests and concerns of your members. As the membership changes over time, these interests will change. Keeping in touch with changing needs is important to the success of your group.

- **Plan routine meeting dates.** We meet monthly on a regular schedule on the same day of the month every month and this helps our members remember when to come.

- **Schedule a speaker or program** at your meetings. It's a good idea to have a speaker at every other meeting. A "name" speaker" or a "hot topic" that is announced well in advance will help attract attendance at your meetings. I try to get speakers who are pretty mainstream and whose techniques are pretty well proven to work, or at least surely proven not to harm.

- **Spread the word.** Use the local newspaper to advertise when your group meets, most papers have a section for support groups and it's offered at no charge as a community service. It's helpful when most of the group uses e-mail. It is an efficient way to communicate about meetings and to share news relating to lymphedema.

- **Welcoming New Members.** Our goals are to be easy going and casual, friendly, warm, and welcoming. New people do not feel intimidated because we care so much. Our members feel good because they are able to help others, and themselves, at the same time.

- **Keep rules to a minimum.** We have only two basic rules within our group. These need to be stressed from the very beginning. They are:

    o **Rule One** - We respect privacy. *"What is said in the group stays in the group."*

    o **Rule Two** - We are not a "pity-party." We have a designated time for "Caring and Sharing" and have found that it is best not to run beyond that allotted time.

- **The Role of the Facilitator.** I am a volunteer facilitator for our group. One of the first things I tell people is that I am not a clinician and the information I give out is from my experience and that of others. It is not medical advice. These words always bring a comment, and a sly smile, from someone in the group who's been there for a while.

Then they'll say, *"But you can count on this information as being good and correct -- maybe more so than what your doctor will tell you!"*

Keeping a group together can be challenging. It can get discouraging when the number of attendees dwindles down to next to nothing (this can happen in the summer months when people are vacationing). I've had a meeting or two where it was just me and one other person, but you know if you can make a difference in that one person's outlook on life it is all worth it. (What! I could be home staring at the TV with my husband!) I can say that I have never resented a minute spent at one of my meetings, even if hardly anyone shows up.

When a group goes on for a long time, you find that some people lose interest. The facilitator shouldn't take it personally because it's a natural thing. After all, there is only so much that can be said about lymphedema!

Usually in another few meetings, new people come on board, or you find a terrific speaker, and they are back again. However, it is a good idea to periodically evaluate what you are doing and to involve the group in the planning process. As the facilitator you need to remember that you are facilitating—not leading—as you encourage the participants to take part in the decision making process.

Suzi Beatie
Facilitator of the Marin Lymphedema Information & Support Group

Chapter 10

Outreach to Medical Professionals

Editors' Note: The stories in this chapter focus on the importance and impact of spreading the word about lymphedema to medical professionals. You will hear from healthcare providers and patients. Perhaps you will follow in their footsteps and educate others, formally or informally.

See also Grand Rounds (page 170) which is a fine example of medical outreach and explains a number of important reimubrsement issues.

I Am a Nurse Educator

"I spread the word and help the nurses understand the risk factors and preventive measures for lymphedema."

Editors' Note: Emily explains how she spreads the word about lymphedema through the healthcare community as a nurse educator.

I am a nurse educator and part of my job is to provide in-service training to oncology nurses about lymphedema. These nurses really care and take their role in explaining the risk of lymphedema seriously.

In talking with these groups I've noticed two patterns:

- Some nurses are not clear about the pathophysiology and preventative measures involved with lymphedema. This is where I come in.

I spread the word and help the nurses understand these factors and how to explain the risk and preventive measures in terms that a patient can understand.

- The second pattern is more difficult to manage. Many of these nurses are frustrated because, although they clearly explain the risk, they know full well that the patient didn't hear anything that was said after the word "cancer."

It is helpful when these nurses have a patient information handout to give the patients to take with them to study when they are ready to hear about lymphedema.

Emily Richter, RN, BSN, OCN

I Am a Lymphedema In-Service Provider

"Healthcare providers really do care and want to be our advocates, but they haven't learned how (yet)."

Editors' Note: Bonnie's experience just goes to show that you can never predict where lymphedema may take you or how much of an impact you may have over time.

I kind of fell into this "in-service" training business. The breast cancer support group at our cancer center (which I don't normally attend) was having a meeting on lymphedema, so I went.

The therapist who was supposed to speak didn't show up; however, the women still wanted to talk about lymphedema. Unfortunately, the facilitator, who is one of the Cancer Center's residence counselors, knew nothing about lymphedema.

After that meeting, I set up an appointment to talk to her and gave her lots of info from the National Lymphedema Network. She was amazed at the implications and urged me to speak to the Nurse Educator on the oncology unit.

It just took off from there. I'll be speaking in early summer to the Patient Safety Directors of about 50 Arizona hospitals and I'm psyched! There's so little understanding—no surprise there—and so much willingness to learn. There are also such open expressions of regret that they haven't known about it and might have endangered their patients' health. It's been an eye-opener for me, too!

I currently use a print-out of patient experiences as part of my in-service presentation for nurses in area hospitals and nurses training programs and they are deeply moved by these voices.

When we struggle with medical personnel, we sometimes think the nurses simply don't care, but in fact they do care—they just have not been educated about this area. The response to this has been unanimous, and this never ceases to amaze me! These people really do care and want to be our advocates, but they haven't learned how (yet).

I'm all for taking this message to the nursing schools, because they're in it for the long haul and they can change the way those of us with lymphedema are treated in every healthcare setting.

As a result of these crazy opportunities that opened up for me, I just got to write an article about lymphedema for the statewide Arizona Hospital and Healthcare Association newsletter. Now I am hoping that will really start a discussion!

Bonnie Pike

Support Groups Reach Out to the Medical Community

Editors' Note: Suzi and Tracy share their suggestions on ways to successfully reach out and engage members of the medical community.

These are only two examples of ways patients and support groups can educate health care professionals. Send us stories and suggestions from your own experiences.

For more information on support groups, see Chapter 9.

The Marin Lymphedema Information and Support Group

"Individuals and support groups can do outreach to educate their local medical community."

Many of us are all too aware that doctors in America are often under-educated regarding lymphedema. For many this is because this topic is not taught in the medical school. However individuals and support groups have a unique opportunity to do outreach in terms of educating the members of their local medical community.

One-on-One: Individuals are encouraged to make a point of passing relevant information along to our physicians and surgeons.

Shared Meetings: The Marin Lymphedema Information & Support Group recently invited a well-known specialist in lymphedema (Professor Stanley Rockson from Stanford University Hospital) to speak at our meeting. Local doctors and healthcare providers were also invited to attend this session and it was a tremendous success.

Suzi Beatie

The West Virginia Lymphedema Network's Show and Tell

"When inviting medical students, let them know that refreshments will be served."

The West Virginia Lymphedema Network support group meets in a teaching hospital. Each year we invite the medical students to a "Show and Tell" meeting.

At this time the support group members volunteer to show the doctors what their condition looks like and tell them about what is required to manage lymphedema.

These are highly successful meetings. One of the ways that we increase attendance is to be sure the medical students know that refreshments will be served.

Tracy Novak

Chapter 11

Reimbursement Policy Issues

Editors' Note: The themes of taking action, educating others, and advocating for change occur repeatedly. If the stories you have read so far have inspired you to join others in working to improve services, insurance coverage, or legislative protections for people with lymphedema, this chapter has facts and resources that you can use.

This section includes:

- Carol Johnson's story of Grand Rounds in two major medical centers covers many important lymphedema care policy issues.

- Results from a patient survey by the Lymphovenous Association of Ontario that illustrate common patient needs.

- Comparison of the costs of treating lymphedema versus the costs, and other impacts, of untreated lymphedema.

- Information on Medicare coverage and appeals.

- An overview of what ASL is doing to help with reiumbursement and other issues.

- Tips for reaching legislative decision makers and tools for activists.

Grand Rounds

"It was inspiring to me to see that these doctors really care about what is happening to lymphedema patients."

Editors' Note: Carol presents her view of the present obstacles to lymphedema care as well as her suggestions for change.

Recently I was honored to be invited to be the presenter at "Grand Rounds" for the surgery faculty and students at one of the major medical facilities in our area. My task was to present information about the lymphatic system, lymphedema, and how lymphedema is treated and managed to physicians who were operating on the body every day!

The lymphatic system has been largely ignored in the medical school curriculums. Again and again, it has been my experience that senior medical faculty and local physicians freely admit that the anatomy and function of the lymphatic system was simply not included in the basic body of knowledge they were required to understand and study. So I was delighted to see a large turnout in the auditorium for my presentation so early in the morning.

Despite normally being a calm presenter, I became increasingly nervous when I was informed by the audio technician that my presentation was being simultaneous telecast to the surgical staff at a second major medical center in another city. However, my nervousness soon gave way to excitement as it was obvious that the audience was very attentive and supportive.

When it came time for the question and answer period, the usual rush for the door didn't happen. These doctors stayed because they had questions and they wanted answers!

Here are some examples of their questions and my answers.

Q: "Why is there such a shortage of qualified lymphedema therapists?"

A: One reason is that lymphedema management in the United States is relatively new. It has only been in the last 20 years or so, that there has been the establishment of a national network of trained therapists. Lymphedema management has not been included in the curriculum of physical or occupational therapy schools, nor is it included in nursing or massage schools. The training for this technique is obtained only by enrolling for postgraduate training in specialized programs.

Another reason for the shortage is because Medicare refuses to reimburse for treatment provided by nurses and massage therapists no matter how well trained and experienced they may be. This recent ruling has cut the limited workforce of qualified lymphedema therapists by at least one third in the United States, creating an even shorter supply of certified lymphedema therapists. Furthermore, because of reimbursement issues many potentially excellent therapists are not entering the training programs making this situation even worse.

Q: "Why is it difficult to get lymphedema treatment appropriately covered by insurance?"

A: There are two major reasons that have to do with coding.

The diagnostic codes used for lymphedema do not begin to describe the variations on this condition. It is much more than "*edema, upper extremity lymphedema,*" "*lower extremity lymphedema,*" or "*other.*" We need codes that more accurately describe the condition. Currently the breast cancer diagnostic code is specific only for women. However, we all know that men also can have breast cancer and a code should be created to describe this situation.

Similarly, the procedure codes do not begin to adequately explain the variety of treatment modalities required to provide appropriate lymphedema treatment. Currently the treatment codes for Manual Lymph Drainage (MLD) must be used to cover all the highly specialized techniques performed by qualified lymphedema therapists. In addition to MLD, this treatment includes (a) bandaging to reduce and control swelling, (b) obtaining accurate measurements for the proper fitting of compression garments which are worn by these patients to control swelling, and (c) the extensive patient education required to enable these patients to provide their own self-care between professional visits.

Q: "You mentioned that insurance companies refuse to cover the compression garments and bandages required for treatment. Why is this so?"

A: Surprisingly, Medicare continues to consider compression garments and bandages as being experimental! This is very likely due to the fact that very little lymphedema research is being done in the United States, even though CDT is considered standard of care in Europe where they are far more advanced in treating and managing lymphedema.

Some plans classify these garments as *"personal comfort items"* or *"not medically necessary."* Trust me, in my many years of practice I have never met a lymphedema patient who would agree with that description!

I have never had a patient request that they be allowed to wear compression garments. They, and their doctor's, know the prognosis for this condition which is chronic and not curable.

Garments need to be replaced every six to eight months. Insurance companies, knowing the expense of these garments, expect patients to pick up the expense. This sets up a roadblock for optimal care since many Medicare patients are on fixed incomes and cannot afford to purchase garments. However, many private insurance companies are partially covering, if not fully covering the cost, as this actually addresses the problem, before catastrophic complications occur.

These garments are medically necessary! Lymphedema cannot be adequately treated without compression garments and denying coverage of these essential treatment aids is like telling a diabetic, *"You have a chronic disease that can be managed so you can live a normal life. However, this can only be accomplished if you pay for the testing materials, insulin, and other medications required to control your disease. Without these your blood sugar cannot be kept within appropriate values and your condition will deteriorate."*

Q: "You mentioned primary and secondary lymphedema and that they are treated in the same manner. Do the insurance companies provide equal benefits for both kinds?"

A: Not necessarily. Under the Women's Health and Cancer Rights Act of 1998 (WHCRA) a woman with breast cancer has certain protection under law including requiring treatment of lymphedema associated with breast cancer treatment. This does not include the coverage of primary lymphedema.

In early 2007, the National Cancer Institute database of state cancer legislation showed that only 21 states had laws mandating that third-party payers offer adequate coverage for lymphedema treatment incident to breast cancer. Of these states, only Virginia requires coverage for all types of lymphedema—not only those resulting from breast cancer. Also Pennsylvania is the only state that requires treatment for Medicaid patients.

When a woman reaches Medicare age, she loses the protection of the WHCRA law. Under Medicare a mastectomy patient is entitled up to six special bras a year; however, if she has lymphedema, Medicare does not cover any of the special garments or bandages required for treatment.

Historically, Medicare has paid for drugs to treat erectile dysfunction, but will not approve payment for a garment that can prevent chronic infection, disfiguration of a limb, and improve the patient's quality of life.

In actuality, it would be more "cost effective" if appropriate treatment was provided rather than waiting for the patient's condition to deteriorate and require more drastic treatment, including hospitalization and even amputation. (See The Cost of Untreated Lymphedema on page 179.

It was inspiring to me to see that these doctors really care about what is happening to lymphedema patients. They are concerned and committed about getting their patients into quality therapy programs, which is instrumental for their long term quality of life.

Bringing about these changes requires the action of dedicated advocates. Concerned and educated doctors can insist that their facilities have certified therapists available for their patients by sending therapists for training. There can also be the establishment of "Lymphology" as a new medical specialty in this country. (This is an agenda item for ASL, see page 190.)

Additionally, and very importantly, the actions of activist therapists and patients can be a major force for positive change. Personally I will continue to be an educator for medical professionals and patients, and support changes in our health care laws that will bring attention to this extremely underserved condition.

I invite other concerned individual to each find his or her own way to also take action to improve the quality of life for those with lymphedema.

Carol L. Johnson, OTR/L, CLT-LANA

Lymph Listens

Editors' Note: Lymphovenous Association of Ontario recently completed an extensive survey of lymphedema patients, breast cancer survivors, and medical professionals. Although some findings are specific to Ontario, many of the issues they identify can be recognized throughout North America and beyond.

Introduction

This article summarizes findings from "Lymph Listens" a community-based study of living with lymphedema in Ontario, Canada. This study was funded by the Ontario Chapter of the Canadian Breast Cancer Foundation and conducted by the Lymphovenous Association of Ontario (LAO) in conjunction with Impakt Corporation. The report was written by Anna Kennedy and Paul Klein. For more information on the Lymphovenous Association of Ontario see page 223.

It is estimated that there are 63,000 lymphedema patients in Ontario. For this study the project team obtained feedback from 150 people representing those with lymphedema, at risk of developing lymphedema, and healthcare professionals.

Of the 115 patients surveyed:

- 92% are women, 84% had breast cancer before developing lymph-edema, and 82% are 50 years or older.

- 80% have lymphedema in an upper extremity.

- 78% had been treated with radiation as part of their cancer treatment.

- The median time between cancer treatment and onset of lymph-edema was one year with earliest being two months and the latest 15 years.

Finding out about lymphedema

Of those who developed lymphedema as a result of breast cancer treatment, 93% with lymphedema reported that they had not been told by any source (family doctors, surgeons, radiation oncologists) about the likelihood of developing lymphedema or what could be done to reduce the risk or delay the onset of the condition.

Only 12% of respondents reported receiving information about lymphedema from any source after they were diagnosed with breast cancer.

In contrast, most of the doctors and nurses who were interviewed stated that patients are told about the possibility of the condition. However, patient receptiveness and timing could be a factor since cancer patients are primarily concerned with more immediate issues such as cancer treatment and survival.

Another factor could be that patients can be diagnosed with lymphedema many years after their initial cancer treatment and therefore any information received would long have been forgotten.

From the perspective of other health care professionals within the community, not more than 20% of patients had been told comprehensively about lymphedema. Instead most of their patients informed them that the focus of post-operative information was on exercises but not on "the risk of lymph-edema," "what to do if it happens," or "where to go for treatment."

After their initial lymphedema diagnosis, 70% of the respondents reported that lymphedema therapists and clinics were their most important sources of information about the condition.

In the longer term, the most valuable sources of information and support were also reported to be lymphedema therapists. This may be due to the ongoing contact that many people with the condition have with their therapists.

Other breast cancer survivors were left to investigate the condition on their own through the Internet, available literature, local health organizations, and with the help of family and friends.

All health care representatives we interviewed agreed that all breast cancer patients should be, "Told about the risk of lymphedema before their surgery to help make informed decisions about treatment options." However, there were various perspectives on when and what type of information should be given.

Level of Knowledge about Lymphedema

Most focus group participants could describe some of the basic symptoms of lymphedema yet were unable to list more than three precautions they should be taking.

There was a variance between those who knew of possible lymphedema treatment options and those who assumed there was nothing that could be done once you got lymphedema.

A concerning discovery was the perception among many breast cancer survivors without lymphedema, that they had been lucky to "escape" the condition and were now risk-free. The lifetime risk of lymphedema was not clearly understood.

Emotional Aspects of Lymphedema

A frustrating challenge for patients with secondary lymphedema is the lack of recognition by the medical community that the condition even exists. Although some patients reported that they were made aware of the condition by their doctors, the implications were minimized—and many were told there was nothing that can be done about it.

Yet the women we spoke to feel their life, as they knew it, was changed forever. In many aspects, the challenge of lymphedema is worse for patients on an emotional level. Cancer has a beginning and an end, whereas lymphedema is chronic and goes on and on. We did not find a lot of focus on addressing the emotional impact for lymphedema patients in Ontario. Although there are many breast cancer support groups that may cover lymphedema information, support groups dedicated to lymphedema are rare.

Cost of Managing Lymphedema

The costs associated with managing lymphedema can be very high. Costs include these elements:

- An initial intensive phase to bring the swelling under control after the initial diagnosis. Average treatment is 12 one-hour Complete Decongestive Therapy sessions scheduled 3-4 times per week over a 3-4 week period.

- Ongoing maintenance phase therapy during which the patient is seen every 4-5 weeks or as needed; roughly 10 one-hour sessions per year.

- Bandages: compression bandaging is worn all day during the intensive, until the swelling decreases and the lymphedema is stabilized. Assume each patient requires two complete sets of bandaging materials. Some patients must continue to bandage beyond this initial phase and will require several sets of bandages per year.

- Compression Garments: at the end of the intensive treatment, the patient is usually fitted for a knit garment to be worn during the day.

A patient should have two of these garments per limb and they need to be replaced on the average of three times a year.

- Compression Aids: at the end of the intensive most patients can be measured for a specialized compression aid, such as a Reid Sleeve, to be worn at night. These garments are only replaced when they are worn out or no longer fit properly.

Editors' Note: Compression Garments and Aids were not separated in the LAO report. See also the Cost of Untreated Lymphedema on page 174.

Barriers to Effective Treatment

Health care providers advised us that besides costs being the largest factor in people not getting the treatment they need, lack of knowledge from physicians play are a great role as well. Patients continually tell them their physician never told them about lymphedema, let alone that there were treatment options available.

High Costs. Unlike most other health conditions in Ontario, people with lymphedema indicated that cost is a significant barrier to accessing the combination of treatments that are needed (in perpetuity) to cope with this chronic condition. Respondents reported that almost all therapies involved costs that are not covered by the Ontario Health Insurance Plan or personal insurance. The high cost of lymphedema therapy and compression products means that many people with the condition simply may not be able to get the treatment they need. Cost of treatment is an even bigger issue for older people, many of whom live on fixed incomes and don't have insurance coverage.

Lack of Treatment Facilities. Diagnosis and treatment are not readily available to many individuals due to locale and a shortage of treatment facilities. One suggestion of the study group is that lymphedema diagnosis and initial treatment should be embedded in every cancer center to equip patients with the proper tools needed for their self-care.

Shortage of Qualified Lymphedema Therapists. Even in large communities, there is a shortage of trained lymphedema therapists. As an example, the Vodder website lists only 45 therapists in Ontario and some patients reported waiting almost five months for an appointment after a referral for treatment.

One of the biggest deterrents for new lymphedema therapists is the high cost of training and certification. This includes the cost of 135 to 160 hours of specialized training, travel and living expenses to attend the training courses, lost income and time away from their current practices.

A recurring theme we heard from our interviews with lymphedema practitioners was the lack of formal or informal networking opportunities for them to share their work on supporting lymphedema patients. Many provided comments that they felt very isolated in a distinct narrow field and that they would greatly benefit from collaboration on best practices, case studies and patient specifics.

Conclusion

LYMPH LISTENS accomplished the specific project goals and LAO now has a clear definition of what is required to meet the needs of those with lymphedema in terms of education, diagnosis, treatment, and financial support for treatment. More information is available from the Lymphovenous Association of Ontario, see page 223.

Summary prepared by Ann Ehrlich

The Cost of Untreated Lymphedema

"It is impossible to place a dollar figure on the cost of a condition, which if left untreated, gradually steals the individual's mobility, productivity, and quality of life."

Editors' Note: We hope that this information helps you advocate more effectively for adequate coverage of lymphedema treatment.

When lymphedema is treated appropriately from an early stage, and the patient is compliant with self-care under the supervision of a qualified lymphedema therapist, the condition can be controlled so that infections are infrequent and hospitalization is rarely required. These patients are able to perform the activities of daily living, to be productive members of society, and to enjoy an excellent quality of life.

When lymphedema is not treated appropriately, it progresses to increasingly serious stages. This progression leads to more swelling and tissue changes that are associated with more frequent, and more serious, infections that require longer and more expensive hospitalizations.

In addition, the patient experiences more pain and becomes less able to perform the activities of daily living. The swelling leads to orthopedic problems and impaired mobility. Many patients become disabled and are unable to work; in many cases family members are also unable to work because of their caregiver responsibilities. Quality of life for both the patient and caregivers decline rapidly.

There are many reasons why lymphedema treatment is neglected as Carol Johnson described in "Grand Rounds" (page 170) and LAO found in Lymph Listens (page 174). Too often the major cause of the failure to treat lymphedema comes down to the bottom line, i.e. "*money.*"

It is impossible to place a dollar figure on the cost of this condition, which if left untreated, gradually steals the individual's mobility, productivity, and quality of life.

Measuring the economic burden of lymphedema treatment turns out to be difficult because:

- Coding issues make it hard to identify all medical claims related to lymphedema (Carol Johnson discussed some of these issues in Grand Rounds, see page 170). Researchers have found wide variations in lymphedema treatment costs and cost reporting due to differences in insurance coverage by plan and by state, and different coding strategies when billing for lymphedema-related services.

- Insurance claims databases only show covered costs. Third party payers do not have data on lymphedema treatment services and materials (including bandages, compression garments, compression aids, etc.) where the patient pays 100% of the cost.

The following cost estimates are based on a study of privately insured working age patients with secondary lymphedema post breast cancer using data from 1997-2002 (see the note at the end for details). These are the most recent figures available and should be adjusted to take into account recent increases in healthcare costs.

Another important factor to take into account is that the participants in this study were all within one year of their initial lymphedema diagnosis. Ideally lymphedema is diagnosed early, before it had time to progress to the later stages where infections are more common and more difficult to treat.

Infection, especially a serious infection that requires hospitalization, is frequently the event that leads to lymphedema being diagnosed. The type of analysis used in this study does not reveal the stage of lymphedema at diagnosis or the sequence of events.

According to this study, outpatient lymphedema treatment during this first year was $1,703 per patient. This figure includes $365 for physical therapy and the remainder in outpatient medical care, all with diagnosis codes indicating lymphedema. This figure does not include the cost of bandages or compression garments required by each patient.

Within this group some patients required hospitalizations for lymphedema related infections and some patients required multiple hospital admission per year. The average cost per hospitalization to treat a lymphedema related infection (cellulitis or lymphangitis) is $9,859. (This average cost is based on all patients with lymphedema, not just post breast cancer.) This cost estimate does not include additional outpatient expenses for infection treatment such as wound care and the ongoing need for antibiotics.

With the passage of time, the cost of professional lymphedema treatment should decrease as the patient learns more self-care skills and requires fewer professional visits. There are wide variations in the amount of follow-on care required; this varies based on the patient's age, physical condition, other diagnoses, lymphedema stage, self-care and support. There are also variations in coverage for follow-on care:

- In Germany and Austria lymphedema patients are entitled to two Intensives each year; each Intensive involves two weeks of in-patient care with frequent MLD treatments, exercise, etc.

- In Ontario (see Lymph Listens on page 174) the expected level of follow-up care is one visit every 5-6 weeks or 10 visits per year.

- Medicare has established a $1780 annual limit on reimbursement for all out patient physical therapy, speech therapy, and occupational therapy. Congress recognized that this cap would harm individual suffering from chronic illnesses, including lymphedema, and legislated exceptions for the year 2006; at the end of 2006 these exceptions were extended for 2007; unless the limits are removed this process will need to be repeated for 2008.

Even with excellent patient self-care, a professional visit is required approximately once every six months to properly manage this condition. At these visits the therapist evaluates the patient's condition and reviews the effectiveness of the patient's current compression garments. If the patient's condition has changed, it may be necessary to measure for new garments. Due to wear, compression garments and bandages that are used daily usually require replacement every six months.

With the passage of time, the cost of caring for a patient who is not receiving appropriate treatment will increase steadily as more frequent infections develop. Continued swelling and infections lead to a degenerative process called fibrosis. Fibrosis is the formation of fine scar-like structures within the tissues that harden and further impair the flow of lymphatic fluid through the tissue.

Fibrosis and swelling create tissue folds that are easily infected and open wounds may develop. The result is that expensive hospitalizations become more frequent and longer. Untreated lymphedema can impair mobility and be disabling, in extreme cases the affected limb may have to be amputated.

Based just on dollars and cents, and not including the value of human quality of life, it is obvious that over the long term it is less expensive to treat lymphedema early and to continue with this treatment including all garments and supplies. Effective treatment can break the downward spiral of continued infections and hospitalizations as we heard from Dr. Stewart (see page 55). In some cases lymphedema related disability can even be reversed and mobility restored as we heard from James Morrow (see page 54) and Liz Pomeroy (page 58).

Until the decision makers understand these basic facts, it is up to lymphedema advocates to bring these figures to their attention and to work toward having policies altered to provide realistic, and in the long term, less expensive treatment of lymphedema.

Ann Ehrlich

Note: Data and cost estimates used in this article are courtesy of Professor Ya-Chen Tina Shih, PhD of the University of Texas MD Anderson Cancer Center and include information from her presentation *Treatment Patterns and Costs of Privately Insured Patients with Breast-Cancer-Related Lymphedema* the 7th NLN International Conference, Nashville, TN, November 2006 and private communications August 22, 2007.

Appealing an Adverse Medicare Decision

"Prosthetic devices (other than dental) which replace all or part of an internal body organ (including contiguous tissue), or replace all or part of the function of a permanently inoperative or malfunctioning internal body organ are covered when furnished on a physician's order." CMS Publication 100-2, Chapter 15, §120

Editors' Note: Mr. Weiss is not an attorney or a physician, and cannot give legal or medical advice. He is, however, well versed in lymphedema matters and has had moderate success in obtaining reimbursements for Medicare patients using the arguments and techniques described below.

Medicare is administered by the Centers for Medicare and Medicaid Services (CMS) to interpret Titles XVIII and XIX of the Social Security Act (SSA) and to implement the requirements of the SSA through a series of publications. Local administration is through a network of Medicare Contractors selected by CMS who either use the national publications or create their own local policies that further interpret the national policy or create policy where a national policy does not exist.

Every service covered by Medicare must be medically necessary and must fit into a "benefit category" defined in the SSA. A specific item is covered if it meets the criteria set up for the specific benefit category, and it is denied if it is deemed not to be medically required or if it does not meet the coverability requirements for its benefit category.

The approach I have taken in appealing Medicare denials of lymphedema treatment is to show that the treatment service or item is medically necessary, that is it is part of a medically recommended treatment guideline and is prescribed by the patient's physician, and that it falls into a benefit category covered by the Social Security Act.

I show that the frequency and duration of Complex Decongestive Therapy (CDT) treatment are determined by a specially-trained therapist treating the patient in accordance with a physician-approved treatment plan. The policies on treatment duration established for rehabilitative therapy do not apply to this medical procedure, and the length of the treatment is determined by medical necessity.

Furthermore, I show that compression bandages, garments and devices fall into the "prosthetic devices" benefit category defined by §1861(s)(8) of the SSA. CMS Publication 100-2, Chapter 15, §120 defines a prosthetic device as follows: "A.   General.-- Prosthetic devices (other than dental) which replace all or part of an internal *body* organ *(including contiguous tissue), or replace all or part of the function of a permanently inoperative or malfunctioning internal body organ* are covered when furnished on a physician's order."

In this case the inoperative or malfunctioning internal body organ is the lymphatic system and the compression items replace all or part of its function.

There are no Medicare coverage determinations or policies dealing with compression bandages, garments or devices used in the function of treating lymphedema, so Medicare Contractors (and healthcare insurers) select policies which deal with materials which look similar but are used in a different function, and apply these coverage criteria for lymphedema. These coverage criteria fail and reimbursement is denied.

Compression bandages are denied for home use because the benefit category they are placed into is "surgical dressings", which are non-durable supplies used in an in-patient procedure in conjunction with treatment of an open wound. This is hardly the function of a short-stretch bandage, tubular sleeve or gauze finger bandage in the treatment of lymphedema! My argument is that the assemblage of these diverse materials every night on the lymph-edema patient's arm or leg is a prosthetic device which is assembled to the exact medical requirements at that time by a patient or an aide who has been instructed in the specific techniques. It makes no more sense to deny a bandage system because its components are not covered than it would be to deny a wheelchair because its wheels or axle are not separately covered. What matters is the *function* of this totality of parts in the treatment of lymphedema that determines coverability.

Compression garments are frequently denied either because they "are not medically necessary" or because they do not meet the requirements of "sec-ondary surgical dressings". The first issue is easy to address by showing that these are different from "support stockings" which are worn as comfort or convenience items, not necessarily with physician's prescription. These are required for daily use as part of the medical standard of care of lymphedema documented in the ISL, ACS, and NLN consensus recommendations.

The second argument is more difficult to counter since 2006, when CMS moved the coding of compression stockings from the prosthetic devices category with HCPCS codes Lxxxx to the surgical dressing category with HCPCS codes Axxxx. The criteria for coverage of a compression stocking as a secondary surgical dressing is that it be used with one or more primary dressing in the treatment of an open venous stasis wound. Denied!

So my approach has been to show that compression garments and devices meet the prosthetic device requirements of the SSA, and are therefore not subject to the surgical dressing coverage criteria. So far two Medicare Administrative Law Judges have agreed and have ruled that the Medicare patients must be reimbursed for their garments (upper limb in one case, lower limb in the other).

A synopsis of this approach which details how a patient can write an appeal is explained in the section below on "Insurance Appeal Logic."

Insurance Appeal Logic

Compression is the mainstay of lymphedema treatment and denial of the medical materials which enable the patient to treat their lymphedema is tantamount to denial of medical treatment. And this is a breach of the insurance contract.

Medicare offers five levels in the Part A and Part B appeals process. The levels, listed in order, are:

- Redetermination by the Fiscal Intermediary (FI) or the carrier

- Reconsideration by a Medicare Qualified Independent Contractor (QIC)

- Hearing by an Administrative Law Judge (ALJ)

- Review by the Medicare Appeals Council (MAC) within the Departmental Appeals Board

- Judicial review in U.S. District Court

I have had some success with the following argument:

1. Lymphedema is a **diagnosable medical condition**, not a symptom. (The medical record should note the appropriate ICD-9-CM diagnostic code.)

2. The recognized **medical treatment protocol** for lymphedema from all causes, primary and secondary is complex decongestive therapy, the backbone of which is **daily compression**.

3. The physician's prescription attests to **medical necessity** of compression materials for this patient. (The prescription must have the diagnosis of lymphedema with the appropriate ICD-9-CM diagnostic code.)

4. Compression characteristics required for day and night are different, necessitating **two different kinds of bandages/garments** (i.e. elastic for active periods-**daytime**, exercise, and non-elastic for inactive periods-**night time**, watching TV, aircraft flights, etc.)

5. Daily use and need for frequent washing necessitates **two sets** of bandages and garments, **every 4-6 months** as required by wear-out and changes in patient's condition and measurements.

6. Compression **when used to treat lymphedema** meets the definition of "prosthetic devices and supplies" in Title XVIII section 1861(s)(8) of the Social Security Act.

7. Compression bandages, garments and devices therefore are **covered by Medicare and Medicaid** as **medically necessary prosthetic devices**. They should also be covered in individual insurance contracts which include prosthetics and orthotics (not all contracts do).

8. Therefore, **denial** of the bandages, garments or devices which are prescribed by your physician for the treatment of diagnosed lymphedema constitutes a **breach of contract and law.**

I help patients appeal denial of compression bandages, garments and devices. It is a lengthy process, taking 1-4 years, with no assurance of a positive outcome, but is worth the trouble because I am using the successful cases to convince CMS to change their interpretation of the Social Security Act and to cover lymphedema treatment materials.

I do not charge any fees for the work I do. I expect that the patient's therapist or provider to appeal the first denial, and when that appeal is upheld (and it will be) then I will help writing the Redetermination Request. For Medicare cases, when that is denied, I will ask to be designated the Authorized Representative and I will write and submit the Reconsideration Request for an "independent determination" by a Medicare Quality Independent Contractor. I will at that time generate an evidence package for use at a Medicare Administrative Law Judge hearing. This is the first level of appeal at which we have a chance of winning the appeal and being reimbursed.

Contact me when you are denied reimbursement.

Robert Weiss, MS
Lymphedema Treatment Advocate
Email: LymphActivist@aol.com

Observations Regarding Medicare Coverage

"Medicare is denying the performance of bandaging under the code for orthotic and prosthetic for numerous reasons…"

Editors' Note: Cheryl Morgan of the ASL has a different perspective on Medicare coverage. For more information on what ASL is doing, see Dr. Tetbar's story page 190.

The comments that Medicare rules only allow PTs and OTs to treat lymphedema are not entirely accurate. The Local Coverage Determinations (LCD) written by each region are reportedly being interpreted differently by the individual Medicare carriers. Not all regions restrict nurses (RN), speech and language pathologists (SLP) or massage therapists (LMT) from providing care—they are mostly unable to bill Medicare under their own provider number and must do so under the supervision of a PT, OT, MD, DO, etc.

Medicare is denying the performance of bandaging under the code for orthotic and prosthetic for numerous reasons across the country. These include: (1) the goals of therapy are not volume reduction but education in self care; (2) bandages are not an orthotic or prosthetic device or instrument; (3) bandages and compression garments are sold to patients over the counter (OTC) with little or no instruction by unlicensed or certified individuals—there is no certification for dispensing these products as there is with orthotics or prosthetics—why then does it require skilled professional services?

It would be preferable to establish codes that are accurate descriptions of the services and products to then secure payment under these codes, instead of trying to stretch a definition of a code to represent something other than what it is intended for.

Concurrently, establishing the criteria for individual education and designation as compression specialists will support the claim that these products are required for comprehensive disease management; require skill to measure for, apply during therapeutic intervention, and educate patients in use. Once these qualifications are established it will be easier to deliver services and procure payment through insurance.

Cheryl L. Morgan, CLT, MS, PhD

How I Became a Phlebo-Lymphologist

"I also began to understand that ... ulcers and other skin infections would not heal unless the edema was addressed."

Editors' Note: Dr. Larry Tretbar, explains how his interests evolved from the diagnosis and treatment of vein disorders (phlebology) to becoming a full-time advocate for lymphology and gives a brief overview of what ASL is doing. For more information on ASL see page 222.

As a young surgeon, more than 30 years ago, I began to realize that lymphedema in the arm following breast cancer surgery was increasing as radiation was added to the treatment program. Lymphedema had been considered a minor problem when simple types of mastectomy were used. I knew little about lymphedema or the lymphatic vessels for that matter.

I also began to understand that a brawny edema (pitting edema and fibrosis) often accompanied advanced venous disease of the legs, and that ulcers and other skin infections would not heal unless the edema was addressed. It became increasing clear to me that the venous and lymphatic systems were intimately associated and that alterations in one system affected the other. Thus I became a phlebo-lymphologist and not just a phlebologist. Because there are many well-trained phlebologists today, I have become a full-time advocate for lymphology. Currently I am also the President of the American Society of Lymphology (ASL).

The American Society of Lymphology continues its mission to support research and educational opportunities in the treatment of lymphatic disorders and to facilitate the establishment of guidelines for treatment, training, information and insurance regulations towards providing optimal care for these health concerns. We are also dedicated to establishing the field of lymphology as a medical specialty.

We have several efforts underway that support our mission and will help obtain reimbursement for lymphedema treatment services and products. These include:

- An improved Staging System that describes the stage of lymphedema more efficiently and improves communication of expected outcomes of therapy and progress achieved. It provides both laboratory and clinical values that can be employed to diagnose, and in some cases predict, the progression of the condition to more effectively develop an appropriate treatment plan.

- An American Consensus Document that is broader than the ISL Consensus Document (which only covers peripheral lymphedema) and specifically addresses issues related to insurance coverage for lymphedema therapy and supplies. This will help standardize diagnosis, assessment, staging, treatment protocols, post-treatment care, and education/training for professionals.

- Creating a process for certifying compression specialists. ASL will be instrumental in standardizing educational requirements for professionals who deliver compression products and assist in securing reimbursement for these essential elements of therapeutic intervention.

- Obtaining a reimbursement code for the bandaging component of the CDP treatment program.

Membership in the ASL is open to patients as well as professionals and all members have the opportunity to take part in educational sessions and to be active volunteers and patient advocates. For more information see our web site: www.lymphology.org.

Lawrence L. Tretbar, MD, ScD, FACS
President, American Society of Lymphology

Advocacy Tools

"It contains very useful tools to arm consumers with skills and resources for change."

Editors' Note: Here are tools designed to help you become a more powerful advocate for change. As Margaret Mead said, "Never doubt that a small group of thoughtful, committed people can change the world. Indeed, it is the only thing that ever has."

When you care enough, and have exhausted other avenues, advocacy or activism may be your best option for getting what you need. Here are some suggestions designed to help you through this decision making process and get you started:

- Define the issue:

    o What specifically do you want to change? Who are the parties involved? What do you want to happen differently and who has to do what?

    o What are you trying to change? Do you want to change a specific decision, terms of a contract, company or agency policy, state law, or federal law?

- Research the issue and your talking points:

    o Understand the parties involved. If the issue is a business find out who are the owners, are they regulated or licensed by the government? If you are dealing with a government agency find out where they fit within the government, what legislative oversight do they receive?

    o Follow the money and look for sources of influence or control. For a business, who pays for their services or how are they funded? For an agency, how are they funded, who controls the budget?

- o   Marshall the arguments in favor of what you want. This should include the reasons, legal or contractual support, costs, benefits, savings or avoided costs, etc.

- o   Make the opposing case and prepare rebuttals. What reasons, laws or contracts, costs, benefits, etc. are involved in not providing what you want?

- Organize support for your position:

  - o   Other people in a similar situation. If this issue affects many people, find ways to identify them and reach out to both individuals and groups so that you can act together.

  - o   Support from your friends, family, coworkers, and membership groups.

- Identify levers and plan actions that fit your situation. Options include:

  - o   Expert opinion and evidence presented via the appropriate channels.

  - o   Media attention on the issue and the organizations involved either as a factual argument or a compelling story. For example, letters to the editor, editorial or opinion pieces, interviews, debates, articles or stories, etc.

  - o   Political pressure on an agency or actions to pass or change laws. Legislators have many ways of influencing government agencies, especially those representatives that serve on oversight committees or budget committees.

  - o   Business pressure: businesses that pay for health care coverage may have the ability to influence coverage decisions or to take their business elsewhere.

o   Public opinion: petitions, letter writing or calling campaigns, picketing or demonstrations, etc. can exert pressure and attract media attention.

Laws, regulations, and policies about lymphedema are established (and can be influenced) at many different levels including:

- National level: federal laws and federal programs like Medicare and Medicaid in the US.

- Regional government (state, province, territory, etc.) level: laws and programs which may be related to national programs.

- Company or organization level for insurance companies and healthcare providers.

- Standards development organizations like the World Health Organization for ICD codes, the American Medical Association for CPT codes, and the Centers for Medicare and Medicaid Services for HCPCS codes.

- Consensus Documents published by various groups are not formal standards but can help define best practice, diagnostic criteria, terminology, etc. There are several lymphedema consensus documents including one originally defined by the ISL (see page 223) in 1995 and most recently revised in 2003 and one currently being developed by the ASL (see page 190) specifically for US insurers.

And to make the situation even more confusing:

- Some organizations play follow-the-leader and rely upon other organizations to establish policies that they adopt or adapt. For example in the US, many private companies follow the standards established by the Medicare.

- Local or regional organizations may modify the policies of the national program. For example, state programs and Medicare regions may have their own rules.

Unfortunately, we do not know of any easy roadmap for locating the organizations or points of influence for each situation. There are groups and individuals working at different levels. For example:

- At the medical policy level, the American Society of Lymphology (see page 190) is developing a Consensus Document covering lymphedema related medical services and insurance issues and has been successful in getting additional codes for lymphedema in the past.

- Influencing policy through legislation and political action are the focus of some groups at the national and state level. For example, The Coalition to Preserve Patient Access to Physical Medicine and Rehabilitation Services (www.coalitiontopreservepatientaccess.org), is working to change CMS policy on therapy reimbursement.

- At the individual level, Bob Weiss advocates on behalf of individuals that have been denied reimbursement, see page 184.

Health Advocacy Tool Box

The Health Advocacy Tool Box (www.cthealthpolicy.org/toolbox/) is an excellent resource provided by the Connecticut Health Policy Project. Although some parts are specific to Connecticut, it contains a wide variety of very useful tools to arm consumers with skills and resources for sustained systems change.

The resources on this site include:

- Tools and Templates,

- Finding and Using Data,

- Effective Communications, and

- Links, including many national ones.

Reaching Legislative Decision Makers

"Making your voice heard is important."

Editors' Note: Are you ready to speak up? Do you want your opinion heard? Follow these tips to increase your effectiveness.

When important decisions are being made by legislators that will affect your health, or on other issues that are important to you, it is important to make your voice be heard. Whether you are a political activist—or an irate citizen who has "had enough" but has never been active in this way before—here are guidelines to help your communication be more effective.

Introduce Yourself!

Each legislator, state or Federal, wants to know that the individual who is contacting them is a member of his or her constituency, i.e., someone who could vote for them when it comes election time. (Special thanks for this tip from advocate Tina Buddle of the Lymph Land website www.lymphland.com.)

Be an Individual

Legislators want to know that this contact is from a real individual—not someone who is casually signing a form letter or petition that is being handed out in a mass movement. To get attention, your communication should be personalized to identify who you are and to state your concerns clearly in your own words. And remember, be concise. Brief is beautiful in the eyes of the clerk or intern who will be reading your communication.

Do Not Mail a Letter to a Member of Congress Because of the anthrax threat, all mail addressed to these individuals is still being sent to a facility in Ohio for irradiation. This significantly delays the receipt of mail.

E-Mail is a Mixed Blessing

In an effort to reduce the amount spam the legislators receive most of them insist that e-mail be sent on an "appropriate" form that identifies the sender. You can send your e-mail directly from the legislator's website.

Be aware that any e-mails not from "the home folks" (in their district) are treated as spam. Also, legislators prefer not to interfere with "personal issues" that are best handled by the representatives of those directly involved. When you go to the website of a senator or representative other than one from your district, the system may refuse to accept your e-mail or it may send you to another site.

Telephoning Works

You may have to work your way through a menu and probably won't be able to speak directly to your legislator; however, staff members are trained to handle these matters and they do keep track of the number of calls that come in either in favor off or opposing certain legislation. Telephone and FAX numbers are usually found on the legislator's website under the heading of "Contact Us."

Fax to the Max

Sending your correspondence by facsimile is probably the most effective means of getting through. Fax is received in a printed form and stands a chance of being read.

Finding Your Elected Representatives

US Federal Government: each state has two Senators and one or more Representatives in the House of Representatives. To find your representatives:

- For the Senate, start with www.senate.gov (notice that this is not a .com address) and look by State.

- For the House of Representatives go to www.house.gov and look by Zip code or by state.

US State Governments: all states have a state Senate and state House of Representatives with the exception of Nebraska which has a single legislative body. To find yours do an Internet search for the name of your state followed by 'State Legislature.'

Canadian Federal Government: for information on your Members of Parliament start with www.canada.gc.ca.

Canadian Provinces and Territories: for government websites start with the Provinces and Territories link on www.canada.gc.ca.

Ann Ehrlich

Postscript

I hope you have enjoyed visiting with the people who contributed to this book. I was thrilled to hear people's stories told in their own words, and to learn from their experiences. It is uplifting to hear from people who are coping successfully and living vibrant lives despite lymphedema.

People express their emotions honestly and openly in these stories. Feelings like anger, sadness, anxiety, worry, self-consciousness, and struggling to come to terms with having lymphedema or feeling overwhelmed at times are all normal reactions. The chapter in **Living Well With Lymphedema** on the emotional aspects of living with lymphedema offers some tips for coping.

Overcoming the Emotional Challenges of Lymphedema explains in more detail how to handle the emotional side of lymphedema. I wrote it because no other book focused on the emotional issues and we heard so much about these issues from people with lymphedema, friends and family, therapists and other medical professionals. If you ever battle burnout, wonder how to answer to people's questions, feel stressed or emotionally stuck, or wrestle with your emotions about lymphedema, I encourage you to read it.

Helen Keller wrote, "Although the world is full of suffering, it is full also of the overcoming of it." The stories you have just read are wonderful demonstrations of this. These stories really bring to life the ideas from **Overcoming the Emotional Challenges of Lymphedema**.

I am especially pleased that so many of the stories shared are examples of effective coping! Many specific stories spring to my mind as examples. Here are just a few.

Actively Taking Charge

Every single person whose story appears here is actively taking steps to care for themselves and improve their lives, physically or spiritually. Many stories talk frankly about the struggle to acknowledge the reality of lymphedema. Others talk frankly about the struggle to find the resources to live well with lymphedema.

Many of our contributors talk about the ups and downs of living with lymphedema. But every story shows a person doing his or her best.

Educating Yourself

The stories in Chapter 3 Learning about Lymphedema] are terrific examples of the fact that the more you know, the better you cope; and the better you cope, the better you feel—physically and emotionally. Over and over, you heard how crucial it is to learn about lymphedema—whether through reading books, going to reputable Internet sites, or finding knowledgeable professionals, peers and support groups.

I give thanks that there are more sources of reliable information nowadays; but it frustrates me that there is still so much misinformation out there, and that so many people have never even heard of lymphedema when millions of people live with it and even more are at risk of developing it.

Finding Solutions

Since lymphedema brings problems, the issue of finding solutions (or alternatives) surfaces again and again. Another frequent theme is the need to speak up or take action in order to get what you need. Sometimes that means persistently asking for help; sometimes it means becoming creatively inventive.

Susan Klapper shares how she builds time for self-care into her family's daily routine (page 138). Avid Gardener (page 125) shares her tips for dealing with the problem of jock itch. Throughout Chapters 4-7 on Activities, Travel, Solutions to Common Problems, and Self-Care Tips, our contributors share their solutions with you. What solutions have you found that you, in turn, would like to share?

Noticing What Works

Tracking what works for you is the foundation for success and a unique example of educating yourself. Learning what works for you and for your body in the special circumstances of your life and your situation, and applying that knowledge, makes you more likely to succeed.

What helps prevent or reduce swelling or infections? Our contributors have generously shared their tips. Whether engaging in backpacking, dragon boat racing, Pilates, pole-vaulting, running, tai chi, water exercises, walking, weight training, or any of the myriad of activities that people with lymphedema enjoy, our contributors try to notice what works for them. One example that stands out in my mind is Tracy Novak regularly recording her limb measurements (page 93). What examples stand out in yours? How do you know when what you are doing is working?

Educating and Helping Others

Many stories emphasize the importance of giving and receiving support. Chapter 9 on Support Groups focuses on this issue. I am especially delighted that so many different forms of support are mentioned.

Sometimes we can even help educate our doctors and other healthcare providers! There are several examples in Chapter 10 Outreach to Medical Professionals and also in Grand Rounds (page 170).

Finding Alternatives

Sometimes you can adapt old activities so you are able to continue them, like Brent moving to a recumbent bicycle (see How Lymphedema Affected My Athletic Activities on page 87). Sometimes you have to find alternatives to activities, like Joanne Young replacing running with walking and weight training (see What I Have Learned from Lymphedema So Far, page 22). As she says, "There are times when you simply cannot participate in certain events or activities." But as the people you meet in this book so often demonstrate, you can find replacements.

In The Joy of Living (page 46) Mary D. Warren talks about, "….adapting to change and embracing new realities." This is just one example of wisdom shared. What other phrases or examples linger with you? What stories will you turn back to re-read in the future?

Facing Fears

Lymphedema can bring fear, anxiety, self-consciousness, and worry. For me, Kim Decker's two haiku poems capture the courage it can take to persevere through the fearful, dark, down days into the good days that can follow, see page 22.

As Audrey's question shows, it can be scary to travel with lymphedema, see page 103. As other stories illustrate, it can be scary to even leave the house with lymphedema when it is visible to others.

Lymphedema therapists can play an important role in helping patients emotionally as well as physically. Plus, as you read in the chapter on Support Groups, going for treatment can provide opportunities to connect with other people with lymphedema.

After reviewing the manuscript for this book, one therapist (Ruthi Peleg) commented on the phrase "education dispels fear" in Fran Suran's story (page 8):

> *I identify myself with this sentence. In order to decrease the fear that new patients have when they phone me urgently to make an appointment, I try to see them the next day. This is in order to reduce their fear and to talk about their edema and the treatment. Even if I can't treat them right away, because I am overbooked, it gives them a feeling of security to know and to understand and they aren't afraid anymore.*

Fear is a natural response to being diagnosed with lymphedema. Yet person after person in this book has found the courage to go out and go on with their lives. You can, too.

Treating Setbacks as Opportunities for Growth

Brent found ways to turn the activities required for lymphedema self-care into reminders and opportunities for spiritual practice (page 136). Bonnie's response to her lymphedema has resulted in becoming an in-service provider, stretching her horizons and offering her new opportunities (page 164). Shelley Barlow is using her body as "an educational tool" (page 18)and Calina Burns is helping raise money for research into a cure for lymphedema (page v).

Finding Inspiring Examples of Success

In the course of writing about lymphedema, and through my work as a clinical psychologist, I am privileged to meet many people who exemplify courage, caring, and wisdom. The contributors to **Voices** are inspiring examples of success for me. So is my co-author, Ann Ehrlich.

Inspiration can be drawn from people you see in the course of your daily life. It can be drawn from public figures, present or historical. It can be found in spiritual or religious texts, biographies or autobiographies, and even through fictional characters who inspire and encourage us.

Ann and I hope that you draw inspiration from the stories in **Voices**. Return whenever you want comfort, inspiration, or advice. Turn to your favorite chapters or stories. Or start over from the beginning and travel again with your companions on your journey of living with lymphedema.

Find ways to live well and join the chorus of voices sharing, encouraging, comforting, and inspiring others with lymphedema.

Take good care,

Elizabeth McMahon, PhD

Appendix

- Appendix A: **Lymphedema Overview**

- Appendix B: **Lymphedema Guidelines**

  o Self Protection

  o Signs of the Onset of Lymphedema

  o Cellulitis Symptoms

- Appendix C: **Lymphedema Glossary**

- Appendix D: **Lymphedema Resources**

  o Books

  o Websites

  o Publications

- Appendix E: **Lymphedema Organizations**

Appendix A: Lymphedema Overview

Lymphedema (LE), or lymphoedema, is edema or swelling caused by an imbalance between the rate at which lymphatic fluid or lymph is created and the rate at which the body is able to move this fluid out of the tissues. The swelling due to lymphedema is skin color while swelling caused by an accumulation of blood, like a bruise, has a darker color.

In lymphedema, excess lymph accumulates in the skin and around the underlying structures. This stagnant lymphatic fluid is rich in proteins that support the growth of bacteria. Any break in the skin that allows bacteria to enter the swollen area has the potential to cause a serious infection known as cellulitis. This infection can spread quickly throughout the tissues of the body and become life threatening.

Primary lymphedema (PLE) is an inherited condition caused by malformation of the lymphatic vessels and can affect either sex. This swelling of condition usually begins in the feet and legs and can appear at any stage of life beginning at birth. Primary lymphedema is more common in females than males and most frequently develops during adolescence.

Secondary lymphedema (SLE), also known as acquired lymphedema, is a condition caused by damage to the lymphatic system. About 90% of lymphedema in the United States is secondary lymphedema due to tumors or treatment. A majority of these cases are the result of cancer treatment, especially when lymph nodes are damaged by biopsy or removed. Other causes of SLE include burns, surgery or injuries that scar or damage the skin, obesity, lipedema, or immobility.

The swelling of secondary lymphedema affects the areas near the location of the injury and the areas drained by the lymph nodes that were damaged or removed. Following breast cancer treatment, lymphedema typically develops in adjacent arm and hand because of damage to the lymph nodes in the armpit (axillary nodes). Swelling may also occur in the chest wall and back, this is known as truncal lymphedema.

Although secondary lymphedema does not necessarily develop soon after the causative event, the patient is at risk of developing it throughout life.

There are preventive steps that these individuals can take to minimize this danger; however, the risk of developing lymphedema does not go away.

Lymphedema affects about 3 to 5 million people in the US including about 20-40% of cancer survivors. The World Health Organization estimates that 170 million people have secondary lymphedema. This includes 120 million cases of lymphatic filariasis (a tropical disease caused by a parasite) implying about 50 million people with secondary lymphedema from other causes.

Although the two types of lymphedema have different causes, the treatment for both is very similar. Currently this is known as CDT or CDP which stands for Complete (or Combined, Complex or Comprehensive) Decongestive Therapy (or Physiotherapy) and includes Manual Lymph Drainage (MLD) to move the stagnant lymph, compression to limit or reduce swelling, exercise to stimulate the flow of lymph and skin care to reduce the risk of infection.

See **Living Well With Lymphedema** for more information on all of these topics, illustrations of the lymphatic system, and much more useful information for patients.

Appendix B: Lymphedema Guidelines

Protect Yourself!

If you have lymphedema, or are at risk of developing lymphedema, follow these guidelines to protect yourself:

- Avoid having a blood pressure reading on the affected limb. The blood pressure cuff can alter or damage lymphatic function within the area.

- Avoid any injection, blood draw, finger prick, or IV placement in the affected limb. Any break in the skin can lead to an infection.

- Avoid having acupuncture needles placed in the affected limb. Although these are very fine needles, they still break the skin.

- Protect the affected limb to prevent injuries, sunburn, or insect bites that can damage the skin. When outside wear protective clothing, sunscreen, and insect repellent.

- Maintain a normal weight. Being even slightly overweight increases your risk of developing secondary lymphedema.

- Wear a compression garment when flying. Changes in cabin pressure can increase the swelling of lymphedema. Also these pressure changes can trigger the initial onset of lymphedema.

- Avoid steam rooms, hot tubs, and saunas. These facilities are designed to raise your core body temperature and make you to sweat. Such heat is best avoided because it increases swelling and could cause the onset of lymphedema.

Adapted from **Living Well With Lymphedema** by permission of Lymph Notes.

Warning Signs of the Onset of Lymphedema

- **A feeling of heaviness in the affected area.** Before you notice swelling, you may notice that the limb feels heavier.

- **A sensation of tightness of the skin surrounding the affected tissues.** Changes such as a ring that no longer fits, a watch that is tight or a shoe that is suddenly too small may be signs of gradually increasing swelling.

- **Swelling, no matter how slight.** Lymphedema can appear "suddenly" as if the limb has ballooned in size; however, this sudden swelling is often the result of signs of gradual increase that have been ignored. Seek immediate medical attention if swelling does develop suddenly to rule out tumor growth, blockage, or infection.

- **Discomfort, such as a "pins and needles" sensation, in the affected area.** Swelling can cause pressure on nerves and this pressure creates uncomfortable sensations.

- **Aching in the adjacent shoulder or hip** can be caused by the increasing weight of the swollen limb.

- **Decreased mobility in the affected joints (wrist and fingers or ankle and toes)** can be due to the decreased ability of the adjacent joint (elbow or knee) to move properly.

- **An infection within the "at risk" area** is often the first sign of lymphedema, see Cellulitis Symptoms on this page. These infections can spread rapidly and be serious enough to require hospitalization.

- **Pitting edema is a diagnostic sign.** To test for pitting edema, press a finger against the swollen tissue. If pressure creates an indentation that goes away gradually, pitting edema is present.

Seek a diagnosis and treatment immediately if you develop any of these warning signs. Once lymphedema begins, it will not go away by itself.

Adapted from **Living Well With Lymphedema** by permission of Lymph Notes.

Cellulitis Symptoms

- A sudden increase in swelling

- Discoloration such as redness or streaky red lines in the skin

- Tissues that feel hot and tender

- Rash, itching

- Pain

- Chills and fever

- A feeling of general discomfort or uneasiness

- Achy flu-like symptoms

Cellulitis is a medical emergency that requires immediate treatment.

Adapted from **Living Well With Lymphedema** by permission of Lymph Notes.

Appendix C: Lymphedema Glossary

Affected Area the part(s) of the body with or at risk for lymphedema.

ALND Axillary Lymph Node Dissection, surgical removal of the lymph nodes in the armpit region.

ASL American Society of Lymphology, see page 222.

Axillary pertaining to the arm pit area.

Bandaging the process of putting on bandages, padding, etc. For lymphedema care, the term wrapping is preferred because it's less clinical.

Biopsy removing a sample for study.

CDP Complete (or Combined, Complex or Comprehensive) Decongestive Physiotherapy, the European term for CDT.

CDT see Complete (or Combined, Complex or Comprehensive) Decongestive Therapy.

Cellulitis an infection of the deeper tissues of the skin that can spread quickly and become life-threatening.

CLT Certified Lymphedema Therapist. CLT alone implies meeting the standards established by LANA; CLT-LANA implies certification by LANA, see page 219.

CMS Centers for Medicare and Medicaid Services, the US government agency that administers Medicare, Medicaid, and the State Children's Health Insurance Program.

Complete (or Combined, Complex or Comprehensive) Decongestive Therapy lymphedema treatment that involves compression, specialized massage (MLD), skin care, exercise, etc.

Compression controlled pressure created by bandages, special garments (see Garment), compression aids, etc.

CPT see Current Procedural Terminology.

Current Procedural Terminology (CPT) a uniform coding system developed by the American Medical Association that is used primarily to identify medical services and procedures furnished by physicians and other health care professionals.

CVI Chronic Venous Insufficiency, see page 72.

DMEPOS Durable Medical Equipment, Prosthetics, Orthotics, and Supplies, HCPCS Level II codes for these items when used outside a physician's office.

Doffing the process of taking something off; opposite of donning.

Donning the process of putting something on; a donning aid is a device that helps with this process.

Edema medical term for swelling. There are many types of edema; Lymphedema is specifically due to excess lymphatic fluid.

Erysipelas a painful infection of the skin and the tissues and lymphatic structures located just under the skin.

Farrow Wrap compression garments from Farrow Medical Innovations.

Fibrosis a degenerative process where tiny scar-like structures within the skin harden and further impair the flow of lymphatic fluid through the tissue.

Fibrotic a descriptive term for tissues that have hardened due to fibrosis.

Fitter a person that has special training in measuring and selecting compression garments.

Garment general term for compression aids designed to fit body parts.

HCPCS see Healthcare Common Procedure Coding System.

Healthcare Common Procedure Coding System (HCPCS) standard coding used by healthcare insurers in the US. HCPCS Level I uses Current Procedural Terminology (CPT) codes to identify medical services and procedures; HCPCS Level II codes are defined by CMS and identify products, supplies, and services not included in the CPT codes, see also DMEPOS.

ICD see International Classification of Diseases.

Inguinal located in the groin area where the lower abdomen connects to the thigh.

Intensive a period of frequent treatments (typically five or more per week) lasting a week or longer and intended to reduce swelling and reverse fibrosis.

International Classification of Diseases (ICD) codes are a World Health Organization standard diagnostic classification for health management purposes. The ICD codes applicable to lymphedema treatment are 457.0 Postmastectomy lymphedema and 457.1 Other lymphedema.

Jovi a JoViPak brand compression garment.

LANA Lymphology Association of North America see page 219.

LAO Lymphovenous Association of Ontario see page 223.

LE Lymphedema.

LMT Licensed Massage Therapist.

LRF Lymphatic Research Foundation see page 221.

Lymph lymphatic fluid, or tissue fluid is a liquid that circulates through the body. Lymph from tissues is collected in lymph vessels, cleansed in the lymph nodes, and returned to the blood circulatory system where is it transported back into the tissues.

Lymphangitis an infection involving the lymphatic vessels.

Manual Lymph Drainage (MLD) a specialized form of very gentle massage designed to move the accumulated lymphatic fluid out of the tissues and back into the circulatory system.

MLD see Manual Lymph Drainage.

NLN National Lymphedema Network, see page 218.

Non-pitting Edema swollen tissue that does not hold its shape if you press and release. Contrast to pitting edema where the swollen tissue holds the indentation.

OTC Over The Counter, medications or supplies that are available in retail stores.

OTR Occupational Therapist Registered; OTR/L indicates state licensure.

Pitting Edema normal swollen tissue does not hold its shape if you press and release; pitting edema is the condition where the swollen tissue holds the indentation.

PLE Primary Lymphedema.

PT Physical Therapist; PTA, Physical Therapy Assistant.

Reid Sleeve a brand of garment designed by Dr. Reid and available from Peninsula Medical Supply.

Short-Stretch Bandage a specialized bandage with only about 70% stretch designed to provide resistance against the skin and muscles.

SLE Secondary Lymphedema.

Sleeve a compression sleeve garment designed to apply controlled pressure.

SLP Speech and Language Pathologist.

SNB Sentinel Node Biopsy, removal and examination of the first lymph node to which cancer cells are likely to spread from a tumor.

Stage clinical term used to classify changes in the skin due to lymphedema.

Stockinette a tubular gauze bandage.

Truncal in the trunk or torso of the body.

Wrapping the process of putting on bandages, padding, etc.

A more extensive glossary with links to related articles is available online at www.LymphNotes.com/gloss.php.

Appendix D: Lymphedema Resources

Books for a General Audience

Living Well With Lymphedema by Ann Ehrlich, Alma Vinjé-Harrewijn, PT, CLT and Elizabeth McMahon, PhD. Lymph Notes, 2005. A comprehensive patient handbook that covers the physical aspects of lymphedema including prevention, diagnosis, treatment, self-care, insurance, nutrition, and much more.

Overcoming the Emotional Challenges of Lymphedema by Elizabeth McMahon, PhD. Lymph Notes, 2005.

Lymphedema by the American Cancer Society. American Cancer Society; 2006.

Lymphedema: A Breast Cancer Patient's Guide to Prevention and Healing by Jeannie Burt and Gwen White. Hunter House, 2005.

Books for Medical Professionals

Lymphedema Management by Joachim E. Zuther. Thieme Medical Publishers, 2005.

Foundations of Manual Lymph Drainage by Michael Foldi and Roman Strossenreuther. Mosby, 2004.

A Primer on Lymphedema by Deborah G. Kelly. Pearson Education, 2001.

Lymphedema: Diagnosis and Treatment by Lawrence L. Tretbar, Cheryl L. Morgan, BB Lee, et. al. Springer, 2007.

Informational Websites

Lymph Notes www.LymphNotes.com offers:

- Informative articles about lymphedema and related topics and stories about people with lymphedema.

- Resources for treatment, supplies, support groups, etc.

- Support via the online forums. There is a separate area in the forums for medical professionals.

National Lymphedema Network (NLN) www.lymphnet.org, see page 218.

Lymphovenous Canada (www.lymphovenous-canada.ca) Lymphovenous Canada has as its purpose to link people in Canada who have dysfunctioning lymphatic systems with health care professionals and support groups in Canada and around the world.

American Society of Lymphology (ASL) www.lymphology.org, see page 222.

Association of Cancer Online Resources (ACOR) supports e-mail discussion lists on lymphedema and other cancer related topics with searchable archives and also provides other cancer related information; see www.acor.org.

Publications

- *Angiology*, a peer reviewed scientific journal from the International College of Angiology and the official journal of the ASL.

- *Connections*, quarterly newsletter from the ASL.

- *Journal of Lymphoedema* published by Wounds UK, see www.journaloflymphoedema.com.

- *Lymphatic Research and Biology*, a peer reviewed scientific journal published by Mary Ann Liebert Publishers, a leading biomedical publisher, and the official journal of the Lymphatic Research Foundation, see www.liebertpub.com/lrb.

- *LymphLink*, quarterly newsletter with detailed articles from the NLN, see page 218.

- *Lymphology*, from the ISL see www.u.arizona.edu/~witte/lymphology.htm

Appendix E: Lymphedema Organizations

These organizations for patients and professionals, including some organizations that fund lymphedema education and care, are profiled on the pages that follow:

- NLN: National Lymphedema Network, serving patients and professionals, page 218.

- LANA: Lymphology Association of North America, therapist training standards and certification, page 219.

- PLAN: Parents' Lymphedema Action Network, for parents of children with lymphedema, page 220.

- LRF: Lymphatic Research Foundation, promoting and supporting lymphatic research, page 221.

- ASL: American Society of Lymphology, establishing lymphology as a medical specialty in the US, page 222. See also page 190.

- ISL: International Society of Lymphology, professional organization, page 223.

- LAO: Lymphovenous Association of Ontario, patient group, page 223.

- NAVALT, North American Vodder Association of Lymphatic Therapy, Vodder therapists association, page 224.

- Susan G. Komen for the Cure, cancer research and support, page 224.

- Cancer*Care*, support for cancer survivors, page 226.

There are many other organizations around the world including:

- Israeli Lymphedema Association, see www.ial.org.il.

- The British Lymphology Society (BLS) a charitable organization with a membership of health care professionals from various specialties, and others who have a direct interest in promoting effective management of lymphedema. For more information see www.thebls.com.

- The Lympheodema Support Network (LSN) is a registered charity and the UK's national patient support organization for lymphedema and promotes the formation of self-help support groups around the country; see www.lymphoedema.org.

- The Lymphoedema Association of Australia, see www.lymphoedema.org.au.

NLN: National Lymphedema Network

"The mission of the NLN is to create awareness of lymphedema through education and to promote and support the availability of quality medical treatment."

Saskia R. J. Thiadens, RN, founded the National Lymphedema Network, Inc. (NLN) in 1988 as a nonprofit organization with a mission of creating awareness of lymphedema through education and to promote and support the availability of quality medical treatment for all individuals at risk for or affected by lymphedema. The goals are to provide education and guidance to lymphedema patients, health care professionals, and the general public by disseminating information on the prevention and management of primary and secondary lymphedema. Membership in this organization is open to all who are concerned with lymphedema.

Member services include:

- Website (www.lymphnet.org) with:

    o   Information about the organization, events, and services.

o   Expert position papers on a variety of topics including lymphedema treatment, risk reduction, therapist training, exercise, and air travel;

o   Listings of treatment centers, therapists and suppliers.

o   Ordering information on CD's, books, videos and specialty items like lymphedema alert bracelets.

o   Information on advocacy, how to start a support group, updates on research; referrals for clinical research; and an extensive patient survey.

- *LymphLink*, quarterly newsletter with articles about medical and scientific developments, information on support groups and meetings, Action Alert and Legislative Corner, product advertisements and lists of treatment centers, support groups, and suppliers. Members may access articles from back issues of LymphLink online.

- International professional conferences every other year and local patient awareness events.

For more information see www.lymphnet.org, phone toll free 1-800-541-3259 or 510-208-3200, or write the NLN at 1611 Telegraph Ave. Suite1111, Oakland, CA 94612.

LANA: Lymphology Association of North America

The Lymphology Association of North America (LANA) is a non-profit corporation composed of healthcare professionals (including physicians, nurses, massage therapists, physical therapists, and occupational therapists) experienced in the field of lymphology and lymphedema. The mission of LANA is to establish and maintain standards for the training and certification of lymphedema therapists.

Basic requirements for becoming a Certified Lymphedema Therapist (CLT) include:

- Successfully completing 135 hours of Complete Decongestive Therapy (CDT) coursework from a recognized lymphedema training program that includes one third theoretical instruction and two thirds practical lab work.

- Proof of completion of 12 credit hours human anatomy, physiology, and/or pathology at an accredited college or university.

- Current unrestricted medical license in a related field: physician, physical therapist, nurse, occupational therapist, massage therapist, or chiropractor.

LANA certifies therapists based on these requirements for education, professional licensure and training in lymphedema therapy, plus supervised experience and a subject matter examination. Therapists who have completed this process are entitled to use the title of CLT-LANA (Certified Lymphedema Therapist-Lymphology Association of North America). This CLT-LANA certificate must be renewed every six years through reexamination or by documented continuing education.

For more information see www.clt-lana.org.

PLAN: Parents' Lymphedema Action Network

The mission of PLAN is to assist parents of young children affected by lymphedema by establishing an active parent networking group, and creating awareness of LE through education.

PLAN is dedicated to:

- Fostering active relationships amongst parents of children that have lymphedema.

- Educating parents on issues related to children with lymphedema.

- Expanding the number and geographical distribution of lymph-edema treatment facilities and certified lymphedema therapists that treat children.

The PLAN website provides information about educational conference calls, recordings of past calls, a message board, etc. For more information see www.lymphnet.org/patients/PLAN.htm.

LRF: Lymphatic Research Foundation

"The mission of this organization is to advance research about the lymphatic system and to find the cause of and cure for lymphatic diseases, lymphede-ma, and related disorders."

Editor's Note: LRF was founded in 1998 by Wendy Chaite who continues to serve as its president. After years of relative neglect by medical researchers, lymphatic disorders are finally getting the attention they deserve. It is the lymphatic system after all, that is the body's first defense against disease. A disorder of the lymphatic system affects virtually every other system in the body. Research into how the lymphatic system works promises preventive and therapeutic benefits for millions of people afflicted with a broad array of diseases.

The Lymphatic Research Foundation (LRF) is a national 501(c)(3) not-for-profit organization whose mission is to advance lymphatic research and to find improved treatments and cures for lymphatic diseases, lymphedema and related disorders. Founded in 1998 by a Wall Street attorney whose child was born with systemic lymphatic disease and lymphedema, LRF has been the catalyzing force in creating national support for this historically neglected area of scientific medicine.

LRF's immediate goal is to increase public awareness as well as public and private funding for lymphatic research. It is only through the advancement of research that improved treatments and cures can be found. LRF's accomplishments have profoundly impacted the field of lymphatic research:

With Congressional support, LRF was instrumental in the creation of a Trans-National Institutes of Health (NIH) Coordinating Committee for the Lymphatic System and has been working closely with the NIH in establishing national lymphatic research programs and initiatives. Through its advocacy efforts, LRF has maintained ongoing Congressional support for lymphatic research and lymphatic diseases. LRF has organized seminal, scientific "think tank" conferences, co-sponsored with and held at the National Institutes of Health and is responsible for the establishment of a premiere, biennial Gordon Research Conference Series entitled, *Molecular Mechanisms in Lymphatic Function and Disease*. LRF is also responsible for the creation of its official journal, *Lymphatic Research and Biology*, an international peer-reviewed scientific journal published by a leading biomedical publisher and indexed in MEDLINE (United States National Library of Medicine). In addition, LRF has funded the first-ever international lymphatic grants program supporting postdoctoral fellowships and has helped establish, in perpetuity, the first-ever Endowed Chair of Lymphatic Research and Medicine at a major academic institution. LRF is working toward the establishment of a National Lymphatic Disease Patient Registry and Tissue Bank to stimulate research and support clinical trials for diagnostic and therapeutic drug development. Patients are encouraged to sign up to join the National Lymphatic Disease Registry. LRF's inspiring and educational video, *Call To Action* can be viewed at www.lymphaticresearch.org Copies of the video are available upon request.

For more information or to donate, visit the LRF website at www.lymphaticresearch.org or contact at Lymphatic Research Foundation, 100 Forest Drive, East Hills, NY, 11548.

ASL: American Society of Lymphology

"Our mission is to support research and educational opportunities in the treatment of lymphatic disorders and to facilitate the establishment of guidelines for treatment, training, information and insurance regulations towards providing optimal care for these health concerns."

The American Society of Lymphology (ASL) is a nonprofit organization and United Way affiliate dedicated to establishing the field of lymphology as a medical specialty within professional health care educational programs in the United States.

Additional goals of this organization are the development and standardization of guidelines for treatment, education and training, information, and insurance regulations plus working to support research and educational opportunities in the treatment of lymphatic disorders. Increasing awareness of the debilitating effects of chronic angiogenic disorders, such as lymphedema and venous disease, creates a greater need for comprehensive and universal standards of care, education and treatment.

Membership in ASL is open to patients as well as professionals and all members have opportunities to take part in educational sessions and to be active as volunteers and advocates. For more information see www.lymphology.org, call 1-800-355-6770 or 1-816- 941-3700, write to P.O. Box 22301 Kansas City, Missouri 64113, or e-mail info@lymphology.org.

ISL: International Society of Lymphology

International Society of Lymphology (ISL) was founded in 1966 and now has some 375 members from 42 nations. ISL activities include a journal, international congresses every other year, post-graduate courses, special programs for young lymphologists, etc. For more information see the organization's web site: www.u.arizona.edu/~witte.

LAO: Lymphovenous Association of Ontario

"The mission to improve the quality of life for those living with lymphedema."

Lymphovenous Association of Ontario was founded as a lymphedema support group; however, its mission has expanded to providing support plus improving the quality of life for those living with lymphedema by raising awareness and providing lymphedema education to patients and health care professionals.

A toll-free telephone line (1-877-723-0033) is staffed by patient volunteers who know what living with lymphedema really means. Questions on where to find proper treatment, fitting of compression garments, and information about the reimbursement process for therapy and garment costs are handled by these volunteers. Medical question are referred to the appropriate professionals. Questions are also answered by e-mail at lymphontario@yahoo.com.

For more information see www.lymphontario.org; this site contains links to other Canadian support groups.

NAVALT: North American Vodder Association of Lymphatic Therapy

The North American Vodder Association of Lymphatic Therapy (NAVALT) is a professional organization of Vodder trained therapists. For more information see www.navalt.org.

Susan G. Komen for the Cure

"Komen local affiliates have the option of funding lymphedema related projects."

Susan G. Komen for the Cure is a very successful fund raising organization that awards grants for research and treatment relating to breast cancer and provides support, education, and other services. For more information see www.komen.org.

Since many lymphedema patients urgently need help, we are sometimes asked, "Does Komen support lymphedema research or treatment?" The answers to this question is "NO" and "YES."

No

The national organization does not support lymphedema specific research or treatment. The Komen mission statement clearly explains, "The mission of this organization is to save lives and end breast cancer forever by empowering people, ensuring quality care for all and energizing science to find the cures."

However, the national Komen office does work with Cancer*Care* (see page 226) through a program known as Linking A.R.M.S to provide lymphedema support and supplies for US patients with financial needs.

Yes

There are approximately 125 local Komen affiliates throughout the country. Each of these local organizations holds fund raising activities (often focused on the Race for the Cure) and up to 75% of net income from each domestic affiliate stays in the community to fund local programs as directed by the affiliate organization. The remaining net income is used to support Komen awards and research grants.

The goal is to meet local needs effectively without duplicating the efforts of existing activities. An affiliate chapter can fund lymphedema related programs if this is one of their priorities. Here are some examples:

- The Mid-Missouri Komen for the Cure affiliate, working through the Ellis Fischel Cancer Center, funded a lymphedema outreach project for educating and raising awareness among rural providers.

- The Komen NC Foothills chapter covered 215 lymphedema treatments for 24 women in their 2002 grant cycle.

- The Maine affiliate has funded several grants that include lymphedema awareness. This affiliate also holds regional workshops to help activists learn how to write grant proposals.

Submitting Grant Proposals

Each affiliate sets its own priorities and accepts applications according to an annual grant cycle. You can find your local affiliate on the www.komen.org web site.

The application form usually provides specific guidance on the types of programs and locations the affiliate will consider. For example, "...breast health or breast cancer screening, treatment, education, or support project." Lymphedema education and screening fits typically falls within these program guidelines.

Also, applicants must be a US federally tax-exempt organization, such as a nonprofit organization, educational institution, government agency or Indian tribe. Many affiliates work with local agencies and programs to maximize, not duplicate, efforts that are already in place.

You may want to make contact with other organizations in your area that are working on, or interested in, lymphedema related projects. By working with such organizations you can meet the criteria for applicants and enhance your efforts and those of the organization you are cooperating with.

When identifying the greatest lymphedema need in your area, be aware that getting funding for garments or bandages (durable medical goods) has a longer lasting benefit that funding only for treatment sessions.

CancerCare

Cancer*Care* is a national nonprofit organization that provides free, professional support services for anyone affected by cancer. Offerings include information, referral, financial assistance, and online support. Patients may be eligible for grants that cover lymphedema supplies.

For more information see www.cancercare.org, call 1-800-813-HOPE or email info@cancercare.org.

Index

About the Editors

Ann Ehrlich is a professional medical writer who also has secondary lymphedema following breast cancer treatment. Ann brings to this book her personal "need to know" on living well with lymphedema. She is a coauthor of **Living Well With Lymphedema** (Lymph Notes, 2005).

Ann is actively involved in the day-to-day functioning of the Lymph Notes website. One of the primary goals of Lymph Notes is to provide current and accurate information including announcements about meetings and lymphedema related events. Ann is always delighted to receive your suggestions or meeting notice and you can contact her by e-mail at ann@lymphnotes.com.

Elizabeth McMahon, PhD is a clinical psychologist with more than 25 years of experience helping patients, many of whom have chronic medical conditions. She became interested in lymphedema while looking for resources for a family member.

Dr. McMahon received her BA in Psychology from Earlham College and her PhD in Clinical Psychology from Case Western Reserve University. She works in the outpatient psychiatry department of Kaiser Permanente in California where she provides individual and group therapy, supervises psychology residents, helps develop best practice guidelines, and serves on the clinical review and quality assurance committees. She is a coauthor of **Living Well With Lymphedema** (Lymph Notes, 2005) and author of

Overcoming the Emotional Challenges of Lymphedema (Lymph Notes, 2005).

In addition to her interest in lymphedema, she writes about ways to increase happiness and prevent burnout and techniques for improving communication and cooperation between patients and care providers. She has a special interest in practical approaches to overcoming life challenges. See www.elizabeth-mcmahon.com for more information and her speaking schedule.

See www.LymphNotes.com for lymphedema information, resources including clinics, suppliers, and support groups, and our online support group.

Other Lymph Notes books—

Living Well With
Lymphedema

The complete patient handbook covering the physical aspects of lymphedema including prevention, diagnosis, treatment, self-care, insurance, nutrition, and much more.

Overcoming the
Emotional Challenges of
Lymphedema

A comprehensive guide for:
- People with lymphedema
- Friends and family
- Parents of children with lymphedema
- Health care professionals and psychotherapists

For more information see:
www.lymphnotes.com/pubs.php/b/voices/
or e-mail sales@lymphnotes.com

Printed in the United States
121542LV00006B/139/A

9 780976 480655